Contents

Introduction

This is a book written to help you with the experiences and emotions you are going through right now, as you keep fighting on through postnatal depression. The illness you have will teach you a great deal about looking after a new life while also trying to give yourself the love and care you need and deserve. While things may feel pretty horrible right now, you can hopefully find comfort at least in the fact that your experiences will teach you things which will stay with you forever, and hopefully make you a stronger mother in the long-run.

The goal here is not to force you to 'battle' anything you aren't ready to deal with, or to tell you about other people who have it worse off. What's important right now is to focus on what exactly is happening to you right now, how you can be supported by those around you, and how life will go on. The goal is to show you that there is a light at the end of the tunnel.

Maybe you haven't quite figured out yet if it is postnatal depression you're feeling right now, and that's fine. This book will have some helpful tips that can come in handy, even if it turns out that's not what you're struggling with right now. And while we can't tell you for certain whether you have this condition or not, we can give you some advice that should be a little more useful that simply telling yourself to 'snap out of it.'

If you're quite certain you do have postnatal depression, then you're one step closer to figuring out how you can start feeling better. You may recognise your own experiences in the ones described in this book, and you may start to feel a little less alone. There also may be some experiences described here that you won't have had, and some experiences that you have had which are not mentioned. That's fine too: everyone experiences life differently, and there is no 'right' or 'wrong' way to feel.

If you're reading this book, you're probably trying to look after a baby right now and can't really commit to reading the whole thing. That's fine! Nobody is expecting you to start on page 1 and read to the very end. Dip in and out when you have the chance, pick and choose your chapters, read it in whatever order you want. What's important is that you allow yourself to access all of the advice you need, and that you do that in whatever way works best for you.

There are many people all over the world who have suffered, are suffering or will suffer from postnatal depression. This means there is a wealth of knowledge and experiences that you can draw on today. Check out the stories we have here, and see what works best for you. Who knows what you'll find out?

A note to the reader

This book provides very general information and should not be used as a replacement for professional medical care or advice. It will work best when used alongside professional care, so if you have concerns about your health we strongly advise that you contact a GP or other healthcare provider as soon as possible.

Becoming Ill

I t's just what you've been waiting for for the past nine months – perhaps even longer if you'd been trying for a while beforehand. Your child is born, often after a very painful and lengthy labour, and a great deal of yelling. And you expect it to be just like in the movies: tears of joy, an instant connection, the feeling that you could not possibly love anything as much as you do this small, screaming human.

But that's not what's happening here. You're lying in bed and not feeling love, or even resentment. Instead, somehow, you feel completely indifferent. How could this be? This isn't how it's meant to happen! You feel ashamed, shocked, even. This is unfair. Something isn't right.

This can happen to anyone.

The scenario I've just described may not fit yours perfectly – it's just an example of how someone might feel when those first signs that something isn't right pop up. If what you're going through is even remotely similar to this, the first thing you need to keep in mind is that this isn't even slightly your fault. Postnatal depression can affect anyone, and there isn't something you've done wrong for this to happen to you.

Many people who experience postnatal depression are coming from entirely happy backgrounds: secure marriages founded on equality and friendship, stable careers, happy homes. You can be an emotional, imaginative person, deeply in touch with your emotions. You may have never experienced any form of depression before. Or none of this stuff could apply to you. It doesn't matter. If postnatal depression is going to happen, it's going to happen regardless of all of these things.

You may have never experienced any form of depression before. Or none of this stuff could apply to you. It doesn't matter. If postnatal depression is going to happen, it's going to happen regardless of all of these things.

What causes postnatal depression?

So you've just given birth to a living, breathing human being after carrying it around in your body for nine months, and you're ready to just get on with becoming a mother.

Suddenly, you're struck down with postnatal depression. Finding out what condition is making you feel the way you're feeling won't answer all of your questions. You want to know why you've been chosen to deal with this illness, of all the people it could affect. And that's completely reasonable.

Why should it now be your responsibility to live with this crushing condition, when you've more than earned your right to enjoy parenthood? Whose idea was that?

Why Me?

Let's get this straight: you haven't done anything to make yourself deserve this diagnosis. Postnatal depression doesn't discriminate when it chooses its victims. It picks members of every part of society, starting several hundred years ago, and affects about 13% of new mothers. This is not something you should take personally or beat yourself up about.

This is something you must accept before you can hope to get better. An illness like this becomes far less overpowering and frightening once you are fully informed. The truth is, we do not yet know exactly what causes someone to develop postnatal depression, though a vast amounts of beliefs and ideas have been explored so far.

Most modern theories can be summarised into three categories: Psychological, social and biological factors. The only idea that has been agreed on by the majority of researchers is that postnatal depression is most likely to occur in those who already have a tendency toward developing postnatal illnesses. These illnesses can interact with other contributing factors to create postnatal depression.

Biological Factors

One explanation for postnatal depression focuses on biological factors, especially on dramatic hormonal shifts during a time when your body is constantly changing.

When you were pregnant, your levels of progesterone and oestrogen will have risen to a higher level than any other time of your life. However, once you gave birth, your body was able to reduce these to the normal amount. While completely natural, these changes can easily alter your emotional balance.

The Baby Blues

Experts believe that the baby blues are wholly caused by changes in your hormone levels. Importantly, however, this is a distinct illness and should not be confused with postnatal depression. You will meet some people who say they've experienced postnatal depression but are simply thinking of the baby blues. The differences will become clear if you talk in greater detail about your own symptoms.

The baby blues hit 3-4 days after your child is born, and generally coincide with the start of your milk supply. This condition will make you feel unhappy, unable to cope and a little tearful for a few days, but you can expect to recover fully in no time at all.

Puerperal Psychosis

It's currently believed that conditions like puerperal psychosis occur entirely as a result of changes in your hormone balance. Puerperal psychosis is a severe type of postnatal depression which can often result in hospital admittance. It's important to keep in mind that this is an entirely separate illness from postnatal depression, and the two should not be confused.

It has been found that there's a very strong correlation in women living with bipolar disorder between childbirth and experiencing manic episodes. Puerperal psychosis (or 'postnatal psychosis') is an extra risk that is added to this correlation, leading to the sudden development of often frightening symptoms such as disconnection from reality, general confusion and hallucinations.

None of this means that women with mood disorders like bipolar depression should never have children. It simply means that the period surrounding the pregnancy should be managed with extra care in these cases, as childbirth can be one of the biggest triggers for mania. Women who have had bipolar mood swings in the past have an almost 50% chance of experiencing a manic episode after childbirth. With this in mind, it's very important that such risks are discussed with your psychiatrist, family and GP in advance.

When the condition is known about in advance women can receive treatment for postnatal psychosis with antipsychotic medication which can stop the symptoms before they become a problem. This is why it's absolutely vital that you and your loved ones keep a close eye on your behaviour during this time. We talk about bipolar disorder, mania and medications in greater detail in our book on Bipolar Disorder.

Thyroid Disease

It is not uncommon for pregnancy to result in thyroid disease. Often, this illness develops in the few months following the birth of the baby, and often fails to be identified. With symptoms which can be easily mistaken for those of depression, such as changes in weight, low mood and extreme fatigue, thyroid disease is quite often misdiagnosed as postnatal depression. If you feel this may be happening to you, you can ask for a simple blood test to check your thyroid levels.

Psychological Factors

The psychological explanation of postnatal depression hinges on pre-existing conditions and is often just as insurmountable and powerful as the more physical causes. The following factors should be considered in great detail.

Depression During the Pregnancy

Some people find that there were warning signals during their pregnancy, which they may have only noticed in hindsight. For example, rather than being excited when they found out they were pregnant, they may have felt afraid, or rather than marvelling at all the different milestones they reached they may have mourned their loss of control over their bodies.

The new ratio of different hormones in your body during pregnancy means crying more than usual is pretty common, but feeling ashamed of your emotions and trying to mask them is more concerning. If you find yourself feeling the need to pretend to feel something you don't, or to hide the things you are feeling, it may be a sign of harder times to come.

In some cases, a new mother can find herself growing obsessive as her due date grows nearer. It can be difficult to sleep, and they'll spend this extra time worrying about, planning or rearranging things. While this could be nothing more than a maternal need to have a perfect, safe world ready for the new baby to occupy, it could also be a sign of insecurity about other potential aspects of parenting.

Similarly, growing apprehensive of giving birth is completely natural – you're preparing for your body to carry out one of the most challenging duties that will ever be expected of it. So while some people will identify this as another warning sign of the difficult times to come, others see it as simply being realistic about a very physically demanding activity.

Importantly, as well as acting as a sign that postnatal depression may be an issue, depression during pregnancy can also contribute to any postnatal illnesses you may get. It can be useful to keep these things in mind.

Personal or Family History of Mental Illnesses

Do you or a close family member have a history of mental health conditions such as earlier incidences of postnatal depression, anxiety disorders or bipolar disorder?

Once you begin asking these sorts of questions, you might be surprised by how many people let you know they've had postnatal depression. If these people are your close relatives, this could be a strong contributing factor for your own condition. Postnatal depression is far more common in those with a family history of the condition.

Where does Personality come into it?

If you have a tendency towards perfectionism and have unrealistic expectations of how parenthood will go for you, you're more likely to develop postnatal depression.

Motherhood for people with this personality type comes as more of a shock, as babies aren't born with your systems and timetables in mind. You will need to place your needs far behind those of your baby, and this means a change of habits, plans and expectations. Realistically (and very reluctantly for some), this will be the case for the vast majority of your child's life.

Social Factors

As with any other part of life, the way in which you interact with society can have a massive impact on your mental and personal health on becoming a mother. After all, no woman is an island.

Poorly Babies

Having a baby who isn't well will increase your likelihood of suffering from postnatal depression. This generally happens as a result of feeling as though you have failed to protect your child, or that their illness is in some way your fault. While these emotions and feelings are completely valid, they're also unfounded. Your baby's illness is in no way your fault.

How's your Health?

Caring for a brand new human being is going to be difficult at the best of times, but having poor physical health isn't going to make that any easier.

Mothers who are already dealing with pre-existing illnesses and conditions will have a whole extra set of challenges to deal with when approaching motherhood. Add to this the fact that giving birth has likely brought about its own set of war-wounds, anything from tenderness to stitches, and the discomfort you will be feeling as a new mother will be unlike anything you have experienced.

Giving birth is a massively difficult physical process which will almost definitely leave you completely exhausted. And having a new baby to cater for means you won't really have time to build your energy and strength back up any time soon. So it really comes as no surprise that a new mother is likely to develop a condition like postnatal depression.

Home Life

As with any other type of depression, postnatal depression can unsurprisingly be triggered by a difficult home life or marriage. During and following pregnancy, these potential sources of instability are just another element putting pressure on your emotions. This is why these things are of utmost importance.

We are currently in an era where family and other social structures are deemed in many cases to be significantly less important than other structures in your life, and where young people are less likely to live near their parents and extended families than previously. Sadly, this means you may not have the emotional support network you need at this time, and may not have the same number of opportunities to discuss your emotions in detail with those who care about you.

This is not to say that society today is unfeeling, or that previous generations were in any way better than the current one. This is simply one instance in which being able to knock on your neighbour's door when you need to talk about your feelings may have come in handy.

Traumatic Birth

Giving birth very rarely goes completely smoothly, but sometimes it goes downright horribly. Traumatic experiences while giving birth can easily create feelings of terror and anxiety, and this can give rise to post-traumatic stress disorder (PTSD). Additional factors like poor aftercare and increased medical supervision further add to your likelihood of experiencing trauma.

While the advantages of advances in medical knowledge and care vastly outweigh the disadvantages, it's not difficult to see why many people mourn the shift from giving birth in the safe and familiar setting of your own bedroom. Hospitals are often overcrowded and understaffed, so they're stressful places to go if you're delivering a package, let alone an entire human being.

The massive amount of strangers and frequent long waits for things like beds and treatment mean that it isn't always the most relaxing, positive place to recuperate from labour. Add to this the fact that trying to comfort and care for your baby can't always be entirely easy, especially while in the hospital. Yes, many nurses and other hospital staff will be completely supportive and helpful, and you won't be entirely sure where you'd be without them, but others can be impatient or might seem like they're judging you, and that can be tough to deal with at this time.

You can try as hard as you like to remind yourself that any bad moods are likely as a result of having been awake for hours, of not being paid anywhere near enough, of being overworked and under-respected, but as you make a third attempt at changing that nappy at 3AM it can be very difficult to take shortness as anything other than a personal attack.

This is an experience common to almost all new mothers, but can feel a whole lot worse if you're also struggling with postnatal depression – and worse still if you've just had a traumatic birth.

The Importance of Knowing Causes

It's vital that you have an understanding and knowledge of things that can cause postnatal depression. This can give you the ability to take a step back and view your condition as something that has come to you, rather than something that comes from you. Doing this allows some people to find ways to deal with it more easily.

Looking into the causes and symptoms of an illness allows you to see which factors apply to you, so that you can piece together why this is affecting you and where the symptoms come from. It also illustrates that the condition is not permanent: it had a starting point, and will have an end point.

What have we learned?

Having postnatal depression is not something you can blame on anyone in particular, least of all yourself. In many cases, self-blame can actually make your condition even worse. This is a condition that can strike women from any background or culture, provided they are of child-bearing age, and happens all over the world. All it takes is having a baby.

We don't know quite yet what causes postnatal depression, but the key factors which have been identified all fall into three main categories. These categories are psychological factors, social factors and biological factors.

These categories are incredibly useful when it comes to identifying which women are likely to suffer from postnatal depression. It isn't possible to determine for certain whether or not you will develop the condition, but it is possible to identify whether you should be keeping a close eye on your moods and behaviours if you seem to be at particular risk. It takes a combination of different factors from across the three main areas to create postnatal depression.

Hormones seem to have a great deal of control over your wellbeing, making them key factors in investigations into the causes of puerperal psychosis and the baby blues. Both of these illnesses also demonstrate the links that exist between physical processes and mental wellbeing. This is also illustrated by the persistent confusion between postnatal depression and thyroid disease.

An understanding of what can cause postnatal depression comes in handy when it comes to distancing yourself from your condition. The fact that your illness has a cause (and therefore a starting point) shows that it will also have an end, and that you won't feel this way forever. Knowing your causes also means it may be possible to alleviate your symptoms by making changes in your everyday life.

Leaving the hospital

By the time you're done in hospital, you may feel emotionally shaken and bruised from your experiences there. This is where you expect to begin returning to normality, but if you find that's not happening for you, you're not alone. For many, the blues that come with the first period of parenthood are very real and very, very persistent.

In many cases, women with postnatal depression don't feel excessively sad, they simply feel low and above all numb. For some, a confidence boost or a decent nap is enough to snap out of this state, but for those with this condition it's a little more complex than that. You'll feel more like an uncomfortable childminder than a real-life mother, and your baby will seem more like a plastic doll than your own offspring. This emotional detachment can be incredibly difficult to process or discuss with anyone else, but it's important you don't allow yourself to become isolated at this stage.

3

Symptoms and Warning Signs

One popular myth is that postnatal depression must be really easy to diagnose, because people just become unhappy and depressed. This could not be further from the truth, because postnatal depression can come with a variety of other symptoms which may cause it to become confused with other conditions.

When it comes to postnatal depression, everyone will experience a unique set of symptoms with no two people being exactly the same – just like any other mental illness. Add to this the fact that people are often oblivious to changes in their mental state and behaviour and beyond knowing that something isn't quite right won't realise that they are having issues with their mental health until they have recovered.

This is why the people around you can make such a difference when you are dealing with a mental illness. Those that surround you will have an objective, external point of view and will find it easier to notice changes in your behaviour. So it's important that close friends and family are also familiar with the warning signs and symptoms of postnatal depression so that they can understand what is happening when something goes wrong.

By the time your child is a few weeks old, it can become painfully clear (if it hasn't already) that something isn't right. This can manifest itself in any number of different ways – anger, oversensitivity, paranoia, etc. Insecurities about your own parenting skills can often lead you to misread other people's signals, allowing you to believe that they also doubt your parenting skills. Concerns about your new, post-pregnancy body can let you convince yourself that your partner couldn't possibly love you.

All of these should raise alarm bells for postnatal depression – if not for you then for those around you.

Watch out for Warning Signs

If it's at all possible, it's best to identify your condition early on, rather than waiting for things to get really bad. You don't need to display every last 'common' symptom to call your condition postnatal depression. If you begin to have concerns about your mental wellbeing, you may consider starting a mood diary.

This often comes in the form of a simple list of the ideas, behaviours and moods you experience each day that you may find worrying. Lots of women with postnatal depression find this an incredibly helpful tool when it comes to figuring out exactly what doesn't feel right. In many cases, people with this illness will only experience a handful of the better-known symptoms, and these can range from mild to severe.

Acknowledging the illness sooner rather than later means you have a chance to equip yourself to deal with it and search for treatment, rather than simply watching your symptoms get worse and worse.

Acknowledging the illness sooner rather than later means you have a chance to equip yourself to deal with it and search for treatment, rather than simply watching your symptoms get worse and worse.

Depression

When we think of postnatal depression, depression is obviously the first sign we'll think to look for, but be careful: 'depression' is simply a blanket term for a set of conditions which manifest themselves in a variety of ways. The simplest and most widely understood explanation for depression is that it causes you to feel sad, either sometimes or all of the time.

In some cases, depression comes with peaks (dizzying highs) and troughs (extreme lows), and the combination of these two polar emotions can be deeply confusing when you're trying to work out if you're depressed. One thing to keep in mind if this is an issue for you, is that in these cases the highs you'll experience will be short-lived, exhausting and unnatural. But there are other symptoms you can look out for which will clarify this further. These include…

- Feeling the world you live in is one completely devoid of hope.
- Feeling like all of the misfortune you and those around you experience are your fault, even when these things are beyond your control.
- Loss of interest and enjoyment from previous passions.
- Reduced libido.
- Loss of weight and appetite.
- Feelings of incompetence, hopelessness and uselessness.
- Annoyance, irritation and restlessness.
- Negative thoughts and suicidal ideation.
- Feelings of avoidance and isolation.
- Lack of decisiveness and concentration.
- Feelings of insecurity and uncertainty.
- Feeling as though you could cry at any moment, or as though you want to cry but can't.

Often, the number of these symptoms you experience will signal the severity of your depression. Although it's only in the past few decades that we've begun talking about depression as openly as we do, it certainly isn't a new condition. Depression is an illness which has afflicted us as far back as records go. Initially, though, the condition was named 'melancholia' by the ancient Greek doctor Hippocrates – a term which was also used later by Sigmund Freud.

Experts in mental health differentiate between mild or moderate depression and 'endogenous' depression, now known as major depression. This original term was used to signal that major depression – unlike postnatal depression – generally stems from within, rather than as a result of a traumatic life event. Mild depression is distinguished from more severe types by the severity of the symptoms, as listed above.

Isolation and Withdrawal

Some common responses to the feelings and emotions that come with postnatal depression are withdrawal and isolation. In many cases, an individual will isolate themselves entirely as a result of feeling unworthy of being a member of society, of a family, or of being a parent.

Often, this is because those with mental illnesses and those who have gone through traumatic experiences find it easier to feel safe within the four walls of their own home, hidden from the dangers and challenges that come as part of life in the outside world.

While understandable, these behaviours are to be avoided if at all possible, as they will often cause a downward spiral in terms of confidence and mood.

Altered Thinking and Obsessive Behaviours

It's often much easier for those around you to notice that your behaviour is unusual than it will be to notice this yourself. This is because with postnatal depression, your thoughts may begin to play on a loop until you're convinced that these things are the truth, and that your behaviours are reasonable. Often these thoughts will focus on dark predictions for your baby, yourself and everyone you love.

Many new mothers find that they begin to fret more about mortality, illness and death after giving birth to a new life, and find this information disturbing or distressing. To make these things even more upsetting, it's possible to become convinced that these thoughts are as a result of an undetected physical illness which will kill you.

It's easy for thoughts like this to lead to feelings of fear and hopelessness, making it very difficult to see the positive and beautiful parts of life. You may begin to feel the need to hurt or punish yourself in some way to try and regain control over your feelings and everyday life. You may also start developing obsessive systems and routines.

Many of these obsessive behaviours may revolve around your pastimes, perhaps leading you to spend more time tidying or cleaning, or thinking about your diet. Often these are ways of reclaiming control over your emotions or another part of your life by pursuing feelings of achievement and satisfaction. However, any positive feelings created through these actions are often short-lived, causing the actions to be repeated over and over again.

The obsessive behaviours linked to postnatal depression are often very similar to those of a common illness known as OCD (obsessive compulsive disorder). However, they can be more difficult to combat in the case of postnatal depression as there is also a baby to look after. Many new mothers can take the idea of taking care of their children to the extreme, worrying that failure to adhere to their strict routine will have dire effects on the health of the infant, or will show the world that they are a bad mother.

Common obsessive behaviours linked with postnatal depression include obsessing over whether the baby is clean enough, whether they're being fed the exact right amount and how hygienic their nursery and home should be. In extreme cases, these obsessions can lead to substance abuse of food, illegal substances, prescription drugs or alcohol.

It's important for friends and family of someone with postnatal depression to be aware that it is possible for certain changes in behaviour to be a result of hidden substance abuse, and to be prepared for this possibility.

The Inability to Bond with your Baby

One of the most worrying, distressing aspects of postnatal depression is a feeling of being unable to bond with your new baby. Much of the distress this causes is because it strikes exactly when you should be feeling the most connected to your baby, so something feels distinctly wrong. Often, sufferers of postnatal depression feel inhumane or unnatural because failure to bond with the child you've been carrying for nine months can feel like the biggest failure of all.

In some cases, women have found that their baby has felt like a frightening alien, and not their own child. This becomes particularly bothersome in the many cases where you're expected to be in close contact with your child, such as when they need fed, changed or comforted when they're crying. It's easy to feel ashamed of the discomfort caused by this, and to become dependent on the help provided by those around you.

Anxiety

Feeling anxious constantly can cause a massive amount of distress and while it may seem as though you are feeling this way because your life isn't going to plan, it's very possible for this to be completely unrelated. Anxiety exists as an intrusive and constant feeling that dreadful things are about to happen to yourself, your baby or someone else you love.

For many people, anxiety is an omnipresent fog that alters every behaviour, thought or decision you make. The condition creates unhelpful ideas which cause you to question your safety and that of those around you. It can often also lead you to believe that you are a bad person or a bad mother, or that you have no control over the events in your life.

What's more, anxiety also brings with it additional unpleasant experiences such as panic attacks – distressing incidents featuring shortness of breath, intense fear and a perceived lack of control. People who have experienced panic attacks tend to explain that during these episodes, it can feel as though they have to fight for every breath.

Feeling Tired?

Tiredness is to be expected in new mothers, but the type experienced by those with postnatal depression is something quite different than the general exhaustion of looking after a new baby. This is a more persistent sense of tiredness, which can't simply be relieved by taking more naps or going to bed early.

This is because postnatal depression comes with an overwhelming sense of fatigue, both emotional and mental. Your usual energy levels can become extremely depleted, leaving you with very little interest in any other part of your life. Apathy can easily take root here, and tasks which once seemed as though they were barely even tasks can suddenly seem completely insurmountable.

In some cases, this fatigue can be easily confused with actual physical exhaustion, and the temptation to cancel your day and retreat to the comfort and safety of your bed can be incredibly strong. As with many other forms of depression, bed for those with postnatal depression can often appear as some type of safe haven.

It's a place where none of the scary, upsetting or exhausting parts of reality can reach you to mess with you, where you are able to create your own rules. It's a place where it's all too easy to pretend you don't exist. This is alright if it only happens once in a while, but if you find yourself in bed during the day too often there is a risk of this habit becoming self-destructive and dangerous.

Unfortunately, bed is also a place where it's uniquely easy to let the world go on without you, and that's the world inhabited by your partner, your new child and any other family members and loved ones. While they won't forget about you, it's common for loved ones to put on a brave face in times of crisis so as not to upset you, which can appear to someone with a mental health condition that they're getting on fine without you.

Often, tiredness can be related to sleep disturbances, and a vicious cycle of daytime naps and nighttime sleeplessness can begin. This, of course, is something to be avoided. But this in itself often won't be enough to drag someone with depression out of the safety of their bed. The exhaustion that comes with depression can be something more immense and all-engulfing than anything previously experienced.

What have we learned?

It can be really easy to misinterpret the symptoms of postnatal depression as something else, especially if you are the person experiencing it. It's really difficult to see yourself with the same objectivity as other people, so a it can be a good idea to make sure people around you are familiar with the symptoms in advance if you feel you might be at risk.

There is no exact set of symptoms that come with postnatal depression. Symptoms can occur in any number of different combinations and intensities. In all cases, however, the speed and success of your recovery is greatly influenced by how early you identify your symptoms. The sooner you identify the problem, the sooner you and your loved ones can begin to work towards helping you get better.

There are a number of key symptoms you may wish to look out for. These include tiredness, withdrawal and isolation, obsessive or otherwise altered behaviour, anxiety, difficulty bonding with your baby and depression. If possible, you should stay aware of the possibilities so you can identify the problem as soon as warning signs occur.

Reaching breaking point

In many cases, sometimes after a short amount of time and sometimes after a much longer period, things will feel like they're too much and relationship might get strained. Arguments can become a common occurrence, often fuelled by the temper and sadness that come with postnatal depression. Behaviour can become dramatic and irrational. It can become essential but impossible to express what you're feeling. Things can begin to get better once you've found a way to communicate what you're feeling with someone you trust, but often will not go back to normal without proper, professional help.

4

Beginning your Search for Help

When you're dealing with postnatal depression, it's easy to feel as though you are no longer part of the world around you. You might feel completely isolated, and this can be really tough. Many women explain that their lives have begun to feel imaginary, and they've had to question themselves constantly. It's feelings like this that make it so important to receive a proper assessment and diagnosis as early as possible.

Being given a professional diagnosis can validate all of the things you've been feeling while allowing you to start searching for the help you need. You won't be able to recover fully until you know exactly what it is you're dealing with. Keep in mind, also, that the symptoms we have discussed are not all the symptoms of postnatal depression, and so are not an exhaustive list of all the things you may be experiencing.

These are simply some examples of what you might be feeling, set out in the hopes of helping you understand that you are not alone and that you haven't done anything wrong. If you feel something is wrong, it's important that you speak with a medical professional, even if your symptoms don't exactly match those described here.

Family and other Loved Ones

In most cases, your friends and family will spot any problems or strange behaviours straight away, but things can be a little more difficult where postnatal conditions are involved. It's extremely common for new mothers to feel ashamed of any negative feelings they have around the birth of their child, and to try their best to ignore, lessen or hide any signs as a result.

Try telling one person you know you can trust to bring yourself that one step closer to getting proper help.

A good idea, then, may be to discuss these things beforehand. Make sure that your close friends, family members and partner are all fully informed about symptoms which might point to postnatal depression. Good communication and honesty are lifesavers in these situations. Yes, the topic can be very difficult to bring up for the first time, but it's absolutely vital you get help and it'll be easier to talk about what you need once the topic has been broached once.

Try telling one person you know you can trust to bring yourself that one step closer to getting proper help. The sooner the ball starts rolling, the sooner it'll reach its destination: recovery. Postnatal depression often comes as a surprise, and it doesn't exactly give you the easiest introduction to motherhood – especially if you're a perfectionist by nature.

Combined with potential factors such as difficult births and complications during pregnancy, it's easy to find yourself wondering if it's all worth it. All you can do in the face of these doubts is challenge yourself to power through, and to look back in a year's time. It's fairly safe to say that, by then, you'll have a very clear understanding of what the suffering was for.

What's the use in hiding?

Pride should not play a role when it comes to your health. Standing up and telling someone you're having trouble or you're struggling with postnatal depression is incredibly brave, so where's the shame? Try to imagine your illness is a broken arm, which stops you carrying out your daily tasks like writing or fixing things. Would you attempt to hide your condition then?

The answer, we hope, is no. If you had a physical ailment, you would most likely tell someone to make sure you got the treatment you needed to get better. Mental conditions can be just as damaging (and in many cases more so) than physical injuries, so why should they be treated any differently? Telling someone you're struggling is the most important thing you can do on your road to recovery.

5

Getting on the Road to Recovery

Eventually, you will reach a point where your difficulties are identified: you are depressed. If you're reading this book, there's a high likelihood you've already reached that point, and are working on getting better. In this case, congratulations! You are already on the road to recovery and can start looking forward to properly enjoying motherhood.

In many cases, clarity regarding the source of your problem will come from an external eye, like a health visitor or community midwife. If this person is a healthcare professional, they will likely be able to identify your condition with just a few questions, though the suggestion that you have depression may come as a shock and take a little longer to process.

The issue with postnatal depression – as with many other mental health conditions – is that it can take over your mind and make it difficult to sense where the illness ends and reality begins. It's incredibly difficult to differentiate between realistic observations and distorted thoughts. This is how a mental illness can really take hold.

The Health Visitor

New mothers in the UK are assigned health visitors, who are allocated following the new baby's birth. The duties of the health visitor begin as soon as the midwife finishes their duties. Normally, this is when your baby is around 10 days old. At this point, the health visitor steps in to record your baby's progress and update their health records at regular intervals.

It's also the health visitor's responsibility to ask the mother the all-important question, How are you feeling? And don't just say 'Fine' to be polite! This is your opportunity to tell someone how you're feeling without needing to sugarcoat anything. You should be able to tell your health visitor exactly how you're feeling without feeling like a failure or like you're being judged.

Mental illnesses are just as serious as physical illnesses. Keep reminding yourself of that. One common concern is that by telling the health visitors about any mental health difficulties, you will risk being seen as a bad mother. Others may fear that they'll be reported to the authority and their child taken away.

None of these things are going to happen, and the unfounded fears you're having are just another part of postnatal depression. Nothing bad will happen if you tell a professional about your wellbeing. They are here to help.

Creating a Recovery Plan

Often, it's a good idea to tackle mental illnesses on a number of different levels, and there are loads of different types of support you can look into. These can include support from health visitors, medication, talking treatments and GPs.

For many, the first point of contact with a mental health support team comes in the form of a meeting with your GP. Having listened to your experiences, they will suggest a talking treatment, medication or a combination of both.

Meeting with your GP

If you haven't been able to tell your health visitor for any reason, another good option is to make an appointment with your GP. If you feel uncomfortable talking to your GP about these things, it's generally also possible to talk to a different medical professional in their practice. Many women also find it helpful to bring a trusted friend to their appointment for moral support.

These appointments can seem scary, so it's generally a good idea to make sure there's someone you know you can trust in the room with you. This person can also help you by making sure you don't forget any important questions if you talk about the appointment in advance, though a simple written list of prompts could also help you with this.

Whether you bring a friend or not, don't worry about getting upset in the doctor's office. If you look at your GP's desk, they will have a box of tissues which you can reach for at any moment. Those tissues will be there for the sole reason that you will not be the first person to need them in that room. As difficult as your trip to the doctor's may feel, it will be more than worth it. You are working on getting better, and this will help.

Where else can I find information?

The strongest and most effective way to begin combatting your postnatal depression is by equipping yourself with all the information you could possibly need. In this sense, we're one of the richest generations ever to deal with this condition. All of the information you need is available to you, you just need to know where to look and who to talk to.

There is a great range of informative books written specifically to help those dealing with postnatal depression – such as the one you're reading right now! There was a time when postnatal depression only existed in a short section of books about other condition. Fortunately, this is no longer the case.

If you can't find the answers you're looking for in a book, there's also a massive amount of information to help you online. Many professional health organisations have their own websites and online databases which can give you and your loved ones free and instant access to everything you could possibly need.

What have we learned?

The first step on your journey towards getting better is asking for help. Sharing your fears, concerns and experiences with another person will help to make the situation more real and let you deal with your issues more completely. A good way to start is by talking to your relatives and friends, or anyone else you feel you can trust. Now is a time to be willing to share and to be honest in your descriptions.

Pride in a situation like this is only likely to increase the anxiety and pressure that are already weighing heavy on you. However, if you explain what you're going through to those around you, you'll make both your own life and the lives of those around you much easier and happier in the long run. If you don't feel ready to talk to a friend, though, there's always your health visitor to turn to.

Your health visitor will be your primary source of professional advice one your baby is born. Keep in mind that it is this person's job not only to care for your baby, but for you as well. They should be considerate and approachable, and ready to hear any news on how things have been going for you. The alternative to this, of course, is to talk to your GP – something you'll no doubt need to do eventually anyway in order to receive the necessary treatment.

Your GP will be able to describe all of the different types of treatment and care that are available to you, so it's a good idea to get this help as soon as you possibly can. The earlier you can kickstart your journey to recovery, the better!

Concerns about Medications

In some cases, the best treatment plan available is one that involves taking medication.

Some people worry that requiring this treatment suggests some sort of failure. They feel as though others are able to cope without pharmaceutical help, so they should also be able to. While this thinking is fairly common, it is also deeply flawed. Try to view antidepressants in the same light you would any other medication.

You wouldn't consider someone with diabetes 'weak' for taking insulin, even though many people are able to produce this themselves. So why would you consider someone with depression weak for taking an antidepressant?

If you find the first medication you are prescribed doesn't work perfectly, don't worry. There are a great number of different types of medications available, and we are still at a point in healthcare where finding the right medication is a process of trial and error. Eventually you will find a medication which offers you some relief from your depression.

6

How You can Help Yourself

No matter what is happening in your life right now, life will go on all around you. This is something that can be difficult to process after having a baby – never before have you deserved a break this much, but that simply isn't an option. If you're struggling with postnatal depression, that's something that becomes a whole lot harder.

Talk about it

Of all the support systems you need to have in place when dealing with postnatal depression – as with any other form of depression – the most important is someone you can talk to. Life will go on whether you're ready or not, and having someone who can act as a link with the outside world can stop you from becoming disconnected and trapped when it seems that the world is moving on without you.

It is best if this can come in the form of a close personal contact, but support groups are also helpful if you don't have this option.

Life will go on

You've just brought a human being into the world, so never before have you wanted everything to stop and let you curl up in a ball as much as you do now. This is understandable. Unfortunately, however, there's now a heap of dirty laundry to deal with, older siblings to ferry to and from school, a whole new mouth to feed. Nobody is going to cancel their birthday, sports day, social event, Easter or Christmas just because you need a day off: Life is going on, and you just have to deal with that.

While you can't stop the world from going around, there are a few skills and tricks that will help you survive your new life with postnatal depression, help you make your life a little simpler to manage, and help you help yourself get better. There is no one answer to making everything alright. As with many other things, the best way to cope with this is to try a whole bunch of different methods and see which work best for you.

Always remember that different things work for different people so if one idea doesn't work for you, just move on to the next one.

Put it into words

This might sound a little odd – you already have loads of words about how you're feeling floating around in your head, why would using words make your difficulties any less difficult? Why would you want to keep a record of something that makes you feel worse than anything you can remember? Well, it turns out that recording your experiences and writing things down can be amazingly helpful for a number of reasons.

We're not expecting you to be the next great poet – the things you write down can appear to be absolute nonsense if that's what happens. What matters is that you're allowing all of the stuff that's churning around inside you transfer onto a piece of paper, and this in itself will often relieve some of the weight that's on your shoulders. Keep in mind, though, that recovery from this condition is a very gradual process, and you won't be cured from simply writing one paragraph.

In many cases, recovering from postnatal depression will happen so slowly that mothers won't know they're getting better for quite some time. However, if you keep a diary of your moods and actions, you'll have a solid and simple way of identifying all of the improvements you've made. If this sounds good to you, try scribbling down even just a handful of words at the end of each day so you'll have some notes to compare in the future.

You don't need to spend a massive amount of time on this journal – just five short minutes of really thinking about your emotions and thoughts will make all the difference. Along with your written notes, consider noting an overall rating for your day at the top. For example, :-(could be a bad day, :-| could be an alright day and :-) could be a good day.

If you do this and take the time to flick through your diary every few weeks, you'll likely see spectacular improvements over the course of a few months. Your notes will also mean that if you have a big dip in your mood unexpectedly, you'll be able to see that this is just a short rough patch and that your overall progress isn't going to be affected. This low mood will end.

Let it All Out

In some cases, a new mother might believe that they are depressed as a result of certain events surrounding the birth of her child. This would make sense, as many of the symptoms of postnatal depression closely resemble those of post-traumatic stress disorder (PTSD). Although the society we live in loves to tell us that giving birth is the most wonderful and proud moment of any woman's life, we also need to keep in mind that it can also be an incredibly upsetting and destructive experience.

Often, a mother who has gone through a traumatic birth will feel as though she is stuck living in the moment of the birth, and this will prevent her from moving on emotionally. In cases such as these, writing it down can be surprisingly helpful. If this sounds like your experiences, try writing down the story of your child's birth from beginning to end, without leaving out any of your feelings, fears or emotions.

Once you've written your story, it's up to you what you do with it. A lot of women have found it helpful to give a copy of it to someone they trust, so that that person can have a much better understanding of their emotions. However, if you don't feel comfortable sharing this personal document, you can simply put it in an envelope and keep it somewhere safe in case you need it in the future.

There is every possibility that, having been hidden, your story will never be read again. However, you will know that it's there if you ever need to re-read it or to show it to someone else.

Master the Art of Sharing

When hidden away, emotional distress has the nasty habit of growing strengthened and magnified with time. If you are able to learn how to share your feelings and thoughts with someone else, that'll be a big step forward in your recovery. Also, sharing is often a two-way street, so talking about your feelings will allow you to gather new viewpoints and wisdom from those around you.

Your Friends and Relatives

Finding some way of talking about your experiences is one of the most important skills you can use in your recovery. Try talking to your relatives, friends and partners. There's no shame in struggling with postnatal depression, so there's no reason you should keep your experiences to yourself. Try to treat this as you would any other illness.

Talking to those around you about your experiences and emotions will give you the chance to take in new suggestions, fresh opinions and any help that's offered. In many cases, this will be someone's first step in their plan to get better.

Learn to Delegate

Talking to other people about your experiences and emotions allows them to play a role in your journey to recovery. In some cases, the people you talk to will want to help, and some might offer to take over some of your daily responsibilities and chores. This will allow you to practice the art of delegation – a learnable ability and skill which can feel uncomfortable or strange to a lot of people.

Remember that delegating, like many other aspects of your recovery, will be a learning process and it may take time to feel comfortable with handing some control to people that you trust. You are not allowing yourself to become a burden by doing this. You are working on building up your character and letting the people who care about you feel useful and valued.

Delegating certain responsibilities allows the people who love you to play a role in your recovery and keeps you from becoming isolated or overwhelmed.

Find a Support Group

A great way of getting input from people who really understand what you're going through is to share your story with a support group. Your first trip to the group can feel intimidating, so it's often a good idea to bring someone with you (provided this is accepted at your particular group). This is also another handy way of staying connected to the outside world, and avoiding becoming isolated.

While participating in your support group might feel uncomfortable at first, many people find that they're eventually able to reel completely at home in this setting. If you are able to surround yourself with other mothers who are struggling with the same condition, it can help to normalise your feelings and show you that you aren't all that weird or unusual after all.

Everyone there will have their own stories and concerns and while it's more than likely that nobody will match your exact circumstances, the group will be able to empathise with different factors and support you in full understanding of what you are going through. Your first visit to a support group will be another massive step forward in accepting the condition as just another part of your life that you will get through.

It's common for people to feel an incredible amount of relief on joining a support group, as they have finally found somewhere they can talk about their struggles, fears and lives in general without fear of judgement. This will be especially true for you if you are able to find a support group which specifically deals with postnatal depression. If you aren't sure where to find a relevant support group, ask your health visitor. In most cases, they will have knowledge of a selection of different support groups that are happening in your area.

If you feel apprehensive about sharing your own story with the group, don't worry. This is a very common feeling, and the group will be understanding of this. You will not be expected to share anything you are not yet willing to discuss. You are only at the beginning of your recovery journey, and these things will get easier with time.

Further information should also be available in your local doctor's office, health centre or library. Failing this, the information you need should be available online. There are a great range of official parenting websites which will have lots of advice to help you.

Recognise that this is a Journey

The language people choose to employ when discussing working though postnatal depression can be very interesting, to say the least. You'll probably hear a lot of talk about 'beating,' 'wrestling' or 'battling' the illness. If this is a set of imagery that works for you, go for it, but keep in mind that imagining this as a brawl suggests that the result will be victory or defeat.

If you encounter a rough patch while 'battling' postnatal depression, it can be all too tempting to give up and accept defeat. Instead, you might try picturing postnatal depression as less of a nemesis you must defeat and more of a road you need to get to the other end of. You stand at the beginning of a long journey full of peaks and troughs, dark and unexpected tunnels, stunning views and slippery patches.

It is impossible to know exactly where this journey will take you, but what is clear is that you're going somewhere. The goal is to make your finish line better than your starting point, and to stay aware of which ideas are true and false while you do this.

There's No Such Thing as Perfect

Often, a lot of the shame wrapped up in dealing with postnatal depression comes from the belief that a good mother needs to be perfect. This kind of thinking can really drag you down. Early motherhood is advertised in the media as a time bathed in a warm, rosy glow, a time filled with wholesome home meals, clean babies and neat homes. But spoiler alert: this isn't what real life looks like. In reality, early motherhood very rarely goes smoothly. Your journey through postnatal depression is the perfect time to try and lower those unrealistic expectations for yourself.

There is no such thing as the perfect mother. There are good mothers, yes, but no two of these will look the same. Sometimes, good mothers are unable to breastfeed and have to use bottles instead, and they're still good mothers. Some good mothers love to bring their tots to things like baby dancing, baby massage and baby signing classes. Other good mothers don't have the time or energy to do this. This is fine, too.

Stop Comparing Yourself to Others

Remind yourself as often as possible that comparing yourself to the other mothers around you won't help anyone, least of all yourself. It'll only serve to reduce your self-esteem, and that isn't going to improve your mood. Also remember that humans are frustratingly good at making other people's qualities and achievements seem much better. Judge yourself fairly or not at all (preferably not at all).

This isn't Forever

Like any other journey, postnatal depression comes with a start and an end. If you forget every other tip you read in this book, remember this one: This experience will end. This isn't forever. Sayings like 'the end is in sight' and 'there is a light at the end of the tunnel' are clichés for two very important reasons: 1. They are true in almost all situations and 2. People are very, very good at forgetting this.

Remind yourself. Leave yourself notes. Say it over and over again. Make this one phrase stick in your mind: This will end.

Changes should be Celebrated

In some cases, a new mother will feel as though she will never be the same person again because postnatal depression has changed some part of her personality. This may very well be true, but is that such a bad thing? You emerge from your journey a more developed, stronger person. Some of the beliefs, feelings and behaviours you experience afterwards may seem strange or foreign to you, but who said new experiences were a bad thing?

Take the Lead

Recovery from postnatal depression is one of those situations where you need to be your own boss. Life is already pretty complicated, so pick a few basic principles and stick to them. Make sure you're aware of what's going on around you, keep your life straightforward, planned and clear, and ensure that you know what's going on in your own mind. With these rules in place, you can begin to feel more in control of your life and will feel better as a result.

How am I meant to make life simpler?!

This sounds like a massive undertaking, but it's far more manageable than it seems. Try to avoid unnecessary situations which make you feel anxious. If you're short on time, ask a friend to collect your groceries, or just order them online. Need a walk? Walk to the shops. Other things can wait. Try not to feel embarrassed when your baby cries in public, if it's something you have no control over.

Simple things like allowing yourself to cry when you need to, or allowing yourself to sit out stressful social events, can make all the difference. If major gatherings feel like they'll be too much for you, try simply inviting one or two of your closer friends to your house for a takeaway or a movie night. We could go on, but basically: don't fill every square inch of your diary. Learn to say no to chores and commitments that make your life unnecessarily complicated.

Learn to plan your own life around the way you are feeling, and remove things that stress or frighten you unnecessarily.

Get Planning

Life can be unexpected, unpredictable and downright chaotic. If things start to feel like they're getting out of hand, it can be a good idea to plan your life through rotas and action plans. Things don't need to get too timetabled and strict, but it can help your mental wellbeing if you manage to keep things clear and simple. Bullet points and wall planners can be spectacular tools when used properly.

Don't aim for organisational perfection if that isn't 'you'. We aren't asking you to change your character entirely, just to sort things out enough for your life to function at a simple, calm level. For example, if you find you've been struggling with limited energy or drive, to-do lists and targets can be great motivation to get working. Make sure these goals are manageable, though! No 'take over the world', please. 'Dress baby and self before noon' is fine for now.

Educate Yourself

Your condition will begin to feel more manageable if you learn all about it! Life is generally much simpler when you know what's going on, so make an effort to enlighten and educate yourself. Look out for books, leaflets and talks about postnatal depression. However, be careful not to over-research. There are loads of chat rooms and forums where people with your condition can share their own stories and ideas. These are mostly a good thing, but can have their downsides.

The main disadvantage to open forums is that people can be prone to turning to them on their bad days, meaning there will be many more anecdotes about bad things happening than there are about good things. It's easy for this to create a very negative outlook for what your life with postnatal depression will be like. These anecdotes will be helpful when you need to know you're not alone in your experiences, but do carry the risk of dragging you into an even darker place.

Instead, focus on making sure you have all of the information you can about coping methods, recovery plans and facts about your illness.

What have we learned?

Doing things to help your recovery is not the same thing as telling yourself to 'get over it' or 'pull yourself together'. It means planning your activities carefully in a way that will aid your recovery and make your life easier to deal with, whatever your mood. It means planning lots of little things which can work together to make your life easier. Writing, for example.

One useful skill you can learn is the ability to delegate and share your responsibilities with those around you. Lots of people who care about you will be more than happy to help, and will be happy that you are letting them play a part in your getting better. Start planning your life so that you can enjoy days that are as unstressful as possible. Create doable rotas and targets so that your life has some sort of direction and structure.

Make sure you know all about the condition you're dealing with, so that you know how best to recover from it. Try to accept that postnatal depression is just another part of your life, and that you will get through it. While you're dealing with it, don't worry about trying to be the perfect partner, friend, employee, mother or wife. Just focus on your recovery, and on accepting yourself for who you are.

All of this includes avoiding drawing unhelpful comparisons with other parents around you. Don't let these insecurities get in the way of getting better. Writing your feelings and thoughts down on a daily basis can help to keep track of your recovery and clear your head in the process. Just reading about a good day you've had recently can make a bad day a little better.

You can also share the things you write with people you know and trust. Sharing is an incredibly important part of recovery. Try talking to your family, friends and other people with postnatal depression, or really anyone who will listen. Support groups can be really useful for this.

7

How to Take Proper Care of Yourself

As pressing as taking good care of your baby is, you can't hope to do this properly if you aren't also taking proper care of yourself. This may seem fairly self-explanatory, but postnatal depression can have a nasty habit of messing with your judgement and causing you to neglect your own self-care.

The Real You

If you're finding it difficult to look after the woman you see in the mirror each morning, it can be helpful to focus instead on the real you – that is, the inner you. This may sound a little odd, but hear us out because this can truly work wonders.

Start by conjuring up an image of what the 'inner you' looks like, for example many people find it helpful to picture this person as a cute little animal that needs cared for, or themselves as a child. Try to keep this character in mind all the time, especially if you are making decisions.

It can also be helpful to choose a photo to represent this inner you – a picture from a magazine or an old photo – or to draw a picture of your character. Try to take note of it every night before you go to sleep, and every morning when you wake up. Redirect some of the care you are giving to other aspects of your life – housework, relationships, etc – onto this inner you.

Eat Well

As animals, we don't simply summon the energy and nutrients we need from the thin air. We can't filter feed or photosynthesise. If we want to function to the best of our ability, we need a healthy, balanced diet. This doesn't mean attempting to count all the calories we take in, cutting out carbohydrates or jumping on any other drastic fad diet that catches our eye.

Eating a good diet means considering the fuel our bodies and minds require in order to thrive, and giving them that. A proper diet like this has the potential to boost your immune system and make you feel better in all sorts of different ways. One tip you should prioritise is to fill your diet with loads of fresh, homemade food featuring proteins, carbohydrates, vegetables and fruit.

Another handy trick is to replace large means with a larger number of small meals, so you can avoid going long periods without eating. This can help keeping your levels of blood sugars regular and healthy, which can reduce the unsettling mood swings you may be experiencing.

While dealing with depression, it's common to be tempted by comfort foods which do very little for us. These may include…

- Chocolate
- Crisps

- Chips
- Fast food
- Wine
- Cakes

Often, eating these treats will sound like the perfect fix when you're hungry, but end up causing more harm than good in the long run. The comfort these foods provide is generally short-lived and once it wears off, it's likely you'll just feel guilty or ashamed for binge-eating or resorting to unhealthy foods. They may taste good, but in reality they offer us very little other than that.

What can I do to make my diet healthier?

Try to eat a good, well-balanced diet, moderate your calorie intake and eat lots of nuts, fruit and proper vegetables – with, of course, the odd treat, (...) There is a lot of discussion about supplements like omega-3 fish oils but, having looked into it, the evidence is quite thin on the ground.

Here Dr Nick Stafford, vice-chair of MDF – the BiPolar Organisation and consultant psychiatrist with the NHS, explains how you can make the most of a healthy diet. The best top when it comes to eating healthily is to avoid any type of 'fad diet' you may come across. These may be stylish, but they are more often than not ineffective and can leave you in in worse shape than that in which you started.

Focus instead on eating a balanced, healthy diet with healthy snacks. Just to get one thing straight: Eating treats like cake and chocolate is absolutely fine every now and again – just make sure it doesn't become an unhealthy habit. Try, for example, getting a takeaway on a Friday, and limiting yourself to that day. This way, you won't feel as though you're missing out but also can't be accused of having an unhealthy diet if you eat healthily for the rest of the week.

Consider planning your treats and meals in advance, to give you an opportunity to think about how you can make each meal a little healthier. Ideas we like include:

- Replace sweets and sugary drinks with fruits like raisins. They're just as tasty and handy, but are much better for you!
- If you need a meal in a rush and are tempted by fast food, try preparing yourself some pasta with sauce from a jar. Delicious, and often even faster than a chippy.

- If you absolutely need chocolate, try preparing yourself a mug of water-based instant hot chocolate, low-fat if possible.

The rules are fairly common-sense: try to avoid foods which are high in salt, fat and sugar, and make sure you eat plenty of fruit.

Get Active!

Exercise is fantastic – I can't say enough about it… Regular exercise thwarts early-onset diabetes, weight gain and heart disease – which people with bipolar are at a high risk of developing. It enhances the beneficial effect of your medication and improves your self-esteem and confidence.

Here, Dr. Stafford expresses his praise for physical exercise. Depression can easily make getting out of bed each morning seem like an insurmountable challenge, so taking some form of exercise can easily seem beyond impossible. But keep in mind that people commonly experience a type of 'high' after exercising. A great amount of research has shown that exercise can be massively helpful to both our mental and physical health.

One such study carried out by Duke University in the US randomly assigned either medication, thrice-weekly exercise training or a combination of these options to 156 adults over the age of 50 who were suffering from depression. After the four-month study, a significant amount of participants in each group showed notably improved mental health: 60.4% of those given exercise, 65.5% of those given medication and 68.8% of those given a combination of the two were found to no longer meet the criteria for major depressive disorder.

Experts believe this may be because exercise encourages your body to release endorphins, a type of hormone which raise your mental wellbeing and mood. So exercising with postnatal depression can be a pretty good idea. Don't be too hard on yourself, but do make a point of keeping in mind that even if exercise really doesn't appeal to you, you should still give it a go.

There is some form of physical activity out there for everyone, just do a bit of research and you're bound to come across something that works. If you want to try working out some of the restlessness you've developed after months of needing to do everything slowly and carefully, running or even a brisk walk could be for you. If you're looking for something a little more relaxing, yoga or swimming could be more up your street.

If you feel you're likely to talk yourself out of exercising, it can be helpful to arrange with a friend to exercise together. This'll make it much more difficult to change your mind about your workout, and may even allow a closer bond to form between you and your friend. Whether you're dealing with anxiety, stress or depression, it's important that you find something you truly enjoy and are able to do on a regular basis.

Ideally, this activity should involve up to an hour of cardio (aerobic exercise) three times weekly. Great exercises for your psychological wellbeing include jogging, swimming, dancing, cycling and brisk walking but if that's not possible, even so much as a 10-15 minute walk each day can have a massive effect.

Relaxation and Sleep

If your sleep goes off-kilter, it's an early warning sign you must pay attention to. If you're waking up early or not getting enough sleep, you need to do something about that, either by reducing your stress levels or doing exercise, which helps. If necessary, take a sleeping tablet early on – don't wait two weeks to do that.

Here, Dr. Stafford explains that the type of sleep you're getting is sometimes a warning sign that you're about to experience a mood swing (especially if you suffer from a mood disorder such as bipolar). Sleep can be a massive area of difficulty for those with postnatal depression, who may end up sleeping too little, too much or a bit of both. It's also a key lifestyle factor which can have strong positive and negative effects on your mood.

In many cases, this can be helped by improving your sleep hygiene, which has nothing to do with tidying your bedroom and everything to do with giving yourself a good bedtime routine. For those with a mental illness, getting a healthy amount of good sleep is essential every night. While this isn't always possible, it's still best to aim for around eight hours of sleep every night. As with many other aspects of care, it's common for new mothers to put a great deal of effort into making sure their babies have a good bedtime routine, and neglect to care for their own.

If you feel you're likely to talk yourself out of exercising, it can be helpful to arrange with a friend to exercise together. This'll make it much more difficult to change your mind about your workout, and may even allow a closer bond to form between you and your friend.

There are a few things you can do to improve your sleep hygiene, some of which we have listed below. This isn't an exhaustive list, but the methods we've included are good ways of getting yourself to think about what works for you.

- Your bedroom is a place for sleep. Try to do anything like watching TV, doing chores, studying and eating to other rooms.

- Bedtimes aren't just for kids. Try to send yourself to bed at a set time each night – ideally not too late or too early – and to get up at the same time each morning. If you have a particularly good night's sleep, write down your sleeping and waking hours and try to copy them the following night. It can take a while to work out the times that work best for you, but it'll be worth it!

- Keep in mind that the quality of sleep you get often comes down to your alcohol and caffeine consumption during the day.

- As tempting as it may be, try not to oversleep. Depression might make it seem like a good way to escape your problems, but in the long run it'll only make things worse.

- Consider your bedroom's temperature. If it's too warm, try opening a window. If it's too cold, try turning on the radiator or putting another blanket on your bed.

Take some 'Me-Time'

Now more than ever, you need a bit of time to yourself to take comfort, but it can be incredibly difficult to find the time to do so. You need to be aware of what's happening around you and your child at all times. But at the same time, it is vital that you find some way of reminding yourself to allow yourself the love and care that you need. Write it in massive red letters all over your fridge, or scrawl it on your hand: make time for yourself.

Keeping in mind how rare a moment of self-care can be at that stage, it's important that you don't waste it on vegging out in front of the TV for hours or scrolling through your Facebook timeline. Do something that will make you feel genuinely good. This is a brief moment of sanctuary in your otherwise busy day. A time for escapism. Try to immerse yourself in an activity which provides you with joy, contentment and satisfaction.

The following are some suggestions of comforting activities you may enjoy, but there are many other things that you might find comforting that we haven't thought of.

- Get stuck into a good book. Pick something that's mentally stimulating, but easy to read.

- Take a movie night for yourself. Watch something with a positive vibe – a fantasy, a beloved classic, a comedy, whatever you like best.

- Get involved in a pastime or craft. This can be something you have enjoyed in the past, or something you want to try for the first time.

- Flick through a magazine.

- Sink into a relaxing bath with bath-bombs, oils or anything else that makes you feel good.

If your low mood is really weighing you down and making it difficult to picture things that would make you happy, try sitting down on a day you feel slightly better and writing that you can use on your lower days. Take a note of anything you would like to try or have already done that you think would make you happy, and why these things would make you feel good.

Build yourself a Comfort Zone

Babies and kids love blankets and soft toys because they provide a sense of comfort and security. This is something mothers could do with learning from their children. You may already have somewhere that you particularly like to relax and if so, that's great! If not, finding one can be really helpful in getting through your postnatal depression. Some comfort zones you might choose include…

- Your favourite armchair

- A picture that you feel happy looking at

- A soothing piece of music

- A book or collection of poems that really soothe and focus your thoughts

- A cosy sitting room

- A soft blanket or throw that you like to snuggle under

What have we learned?

As important as it is that you take care of your new baby and other people in your life, this should never take away from the care you give yourself. If you find caring for yourself difficult, imagine a separate, 'inner' you that you can focus your love on.

Introducing some gentle exercise to your daily routine can make your body produce endorphins, hormones which make you feel good. As unpleasant as this may sound initially, it'll get easier over time and will have a wonderful impact on your mental and physical health.

Take on little hobbies and things that will bring you reassurance and peace. Make sure you have 'you time' every now and then, and to fill this time with the things you like. Giving your inner self all of the self care it needs will make your journey to health a far simpler, smoother road. Try to improve your sleep hygiene for a healthier sleep and rest routine. Begin by making sure you don't use your bedroom for anything other than sleeping – no eating, studying or ironing, please!

Try to keep your diet as healthy as possible to give your body the best chance of fighting through the day. Try to avoid too many snacks or junk food.

8

Dealing with Your New Role as a Mother

f you're worried that your postnatal depression will have a negative impact on your baby's health, that's understandable. You're currently trying to deal with some pretty dark feelings while trying to provide a new, tiny human with a healthy upbringing. That sounds pretty difficult! But how will your postnatal depression really affect your baby, and is there anything to do to make things better?

Firstly, as we've no doubt said over and over again over the course of this book, struggling with postnatal depression doesn't mean you're a bad mother in any way. This isn't your fault at all, so it doesn't reflect on your character. If you take on all of the tips and help that are available to you, not only will you recover, but you will become a spectacular mother.

If you leave your postnatal depression untreated, medical experts believe it is possible for your child to be affected in the following ways.

- It is possible for there to be a sense of detachment between the baby and its mother as the baby learns and grows.

- Babies who have limited contact with their mothers are sometimes slower to develop certain educational and life skills, such as speech.

- As a child, your baby may be less emotionally secure than most.

None of these should be perceived as reasons to blame yourself for either your postnatal depression or your baby's development. Always remember that babies have a very limited sense of deep emotions.

Transferring your Feelings onto your Child

It is common for those who feel emotionally drained or vulnerable to unwittingly transfer their own feelings onto those around them. In your case, this may be your baby. In your situation, it's common to worry that your baby is refusing to sleep because your moods are upsetting them, or that they're crying because they're miserable around you.

Many mothers find themselves imagining that they are able to sense how their baby is feeling, but this isn't the case. They're simply transferring their own concerns onto an infant who has no understanding of their condition or mood. On bad days, a mother with postnatal depression may go so far as to believe things like 'the baby knows I need to sleep, so he's intentionally refusing to settle' or 'the baby is crying just to spite me.'

We know that you know your baby hasn't developed the concepts of malice or spite yet. They're simply being a baby who has no means of communication beyond crying, and very little sense of anything beyond their love for their mother. You and your baby must be there for each other, because your conditions are inextricably linked.

Becoming a Mother

People seem to be very keen on claiming that the second you give birth, your motherly instincts will kick in and you'll instantly know exactly what you need to do to raise this child perfectly. This, shockingly, is not the case. The only thing giving birth does is prove that you're capable of reproducing. Mothering skills come later – just like your newborn baby, you're currently just a newborn mother.

The myth of instant motherhood has been passed down through the generations, and as a result has caused mothers endless amounts of insecurity and stress from generation to generation. In some cases, the overwhelming sense of all-consuming motherly love and care just doesn't happen straight away. Maybe giving birth has just left you feeling numb, empty, completely detached from your baby.

Love will come eventually, but it doesn't just happen the second the baby is out. Like most things, it's something that happens gradually, and that's just fine.

Do it all Your Way

To be a good parent, there is one box you need to tick: you need to look after your child as well as you possibly can. That's it. There's nothing in the rulebook about doing what others say you should be doing, or about doing what's popular on Pinterest. You just need to do whatever you feel is best for your baby.

For this reason, it's often a good idea to avoid websites and books about how you should go about parenting. These often only serve to make new mothers feel inept and insecure. There are likely more books and opinionated people and judgy forum-goers out there than there are babies. Yes, these books and websites can be handy when you need advice about specific issues, but that's all they should be used for. Don't read them from cover to cover and attempt to follow them to the letter, as this will often only make you feel inadequate or low when your baby doesn't respond to a certain thing

Most importantly, do what feels right for your baby, your circumstances and yourself. And when you do this, try to be confident and stick by your decision, because it's more than likely the right call. You don't need to try and justify every decision you make to random people on the internet.

> Love will come eventually, but it doesn't just happen the second the baby is out. Like most things, it's something that happens gradually, and that's just fine.

Sometimes, mothers are made to feel humiliated, inadequate or ashamed if they choose not to breastfeed, or if they are unable to for any reason. If this applies to you, don't let it! Your decision is your own, and is completely valid. Understand that this is your choice, your child and your body, and nobody else should have a say in this matter.

Simplify your Life

If you're able to make life easier for yourself, you'll be able to spend more time focusing on yourself and your baby. You're already trying to cope with an unfair situation, there's nothing wrong with trying to simplify things a little.

Get into a Routine

It's likely you'll also find your life easier to manage if you introduce some type of routine as well. This will reduce the amount of stress in your life, and create a sense of security for both you and your child.

Babies love living life as part of a routine. It means they have some idea of what to expect, be it bedtime, play or a feed. It's likely you'll also find your life easier to manage if you introduce some type of routine as well. This will reduce the amount of stress in your life, and create a sense of security for both you and your child.

Take things one day at a time

Just one day of caring for your baby can feel like an impossible task, and it's easy to find yourself worrying about how you're going to survive for a whole week. The solution to this is to stop looking so far ahead. Take things one hour, one day, one activity at a time. Like many other aspects of your life, this will get easier if you try breaking it down into more manageable sections.

Plan in Advance

As much as is possible, make sure you're fully prepared before initiating any sort of feed, nappy change or bath. Write yourself a list of everything you need to have to hand, even if lists aren't normally your thing, and follow it. This will be a great way of keeping your thoughts organised and clear, avoiding the confusion that often comes with postnatal depression.

That said, it's important you don't end up making your life overly complicated with too many lists. Only use so many lists as are helpful in making life easier and simpler for you and your family.

Create a Safe Space

If you feel it's necessary, don't be afraid to take sanctuary with your baby and shut the rest of the world away (for a short time). Create a space where it's comfortable and safe for you to do this. Make it clear that – for a short time at least – you don't want any visitors, and don't feel obligated to take any phonecalls.

Early motherhood is one of the very few times where it's completely socially acceptable to disappear into your home with your baby and partner, because it's a time when you need to focus on yourself and your family.

'Good Enough' is good enough

There is no such thing as perfection when it comes to motherhood, so stop kicking yourself for 'only' being 'good enough.' Looking after a baby is hectic, exhausting and sometimes almost impossible. The goal for any parent is to be 'good enough,' and to accept that that's as close as anyone will get to perfect.

Accept that your baby isn't going to be perfectly dressed, bathed and ready to go by noon. Just having a healthy, happy and fed baby when it comes to teatime is enough for you to call yourself a wonderful mum.

Sleep when your baby sleeps

It may seem a little odd, but it makes a great amount of sense when you think about it. If you're sleep deprived – like most other new mothers – you need to catch up on your sleep somehow if you want to function to the best of your ability. The easiest way to do this is to grab a nap whenever your baby does.

Getting a little extra sleep whenever possible will improve your mood and calm you down, allowing you to deal with all of the little dramas motherhood will hit you with far more easily. It can be tempting to try and get chores done while your baby sleeps – when else will you get the chance? But it's far more important that you get the sleep you need if you want to recover.

Share the Load

You don't need to be the sole provider and caregiver for your baby to be an amazing mother. You just need to learn how to delegate properly. If you're able to take a break from childcare every once in a while, the time you do spend caring for your baby will become far more special, not to mention more manageable. It also means you'll have more time to yourself where you can focus on looking after your own wellbeing.

Don't feel like you're bothering people if you ask them to look after your baby for a time: relatives and friends will always be thrilled to help. Having a baby to spoil and look after for a day isn't a daily chore, as it is when you have your own infant, but a novelty which they've probably been looking forward to since they first heard you were pregnant.

Never hesitate to ask for help if you need it.

Part-Time Childcare

Another option for reliable childcare comes in the form of schemes and volunteers which are made available for new mothers like yourself.

Outside help from places like day nurseries can be a godsend for new parents, even if it's only for a couple of hours each week. Your baby will receive proper, professional care, and will even gain added benefits from higher levels of social interaction. What's more, you will be able to take a quick break from motherhood and return more loving and refreshed than ever before.

Local and Government Schemes

Another option for reliable childcare comes in the form of schemes and volunteers which are made available for new mothers like yourself. Schemes like this are designed with your baby's wellbeing and development in mind, often taking the form of volunteers who happily spend just a few hours every week doing things that will make life easier for you. Look into schemes like www.home-start.org.uk which have branches all over the UK ready to help people like you.

What have we learned?

One of the main worries new mothers have regarding their postnatal depression is whether it can have an adverse effect on their baby. But if you seek help early enough in your condition, any negative affects can be reduced or avoided entirely. The best way of bringing up a baby is to do whatever feels right to you as its mother. Medical professionals aside, nobody will know all that much more than you do.

Get lots of other people involved in your baby's care. Increased social interaction will only serve to improve your baby's development, and you need all the rest you can get. If you deal with your condition effectively, there's every likelihood postnatal depression won't negatively influence your baby's development or health. Take control of your illness, and you'll make things better for the both of you.

Try to make life as simple for yourself and your baby as you possibly can. There's nothing wrong with taking all the help and shortcuts you need to make your life organised and easy. For now, a simple life is a happy one. Relaxation, security and routine will be immensely helpful in this respect.

Even if the universe seems to be working against you, there are loads of ways you can give your baby the best possible start in life. The most important thing to keep in mind is that the idea of instantly becoming an amazing mother is completely imaginary. Being a good mother is a skill that you have to learn, just like riding a bike. And any emotions that appear to be missing initially will arrive in time.

9

How you can help a relative or loved one with postnatal depression (and how to look after yourself)

Often, the people who love us the most will have the hardest time when we suffer from mental illnesses, and this is no less the case for postnatal depression than any other condition. It can be pretty rare for the partner of someone with postnatal depression to be asked how they are coping with the situation, as it might feel a little insensitive to acknowledge that these times are tough for people other than the mother.

Unfortunately, it's very common for mother-in-laws, friends, grandmothers and fathers (and anyone else who finds someone close to them suffering) to become neglected at this time. They can be struggling with their own problems, but they'll still happily be supportive and loyal to the people they love. This chapter hopes to help anyone who is helping a loved one through postnatal depression – parents, husbands, friends and anyone else this applies to.

We've put together some quick tips for how you can provide better care to someone with postnatal depression, without adversely impacting your own wellbeing. Just like the new mother, you need to consider ways you can make your own life healthier and easier, because being a good carer means caring for yourself as well as others.

What are we dealing with here?

Being a carer is one of the situations where ignorance is definitely not bliss, so it's important you know what you're up against when a loved one is dealing with postnatal depression. It's likely that you're already acquainted with some of the better-known symptoms of this condition, but there will probably also be some more subtle symptoms of which you aren't aware.

You may notice certain new behaviours that are different from the sufferer's usual behaviour, and this can be upsetting. In these cases, knowing that they're simply a symptom of their illness can be a real reassurance. If you're reading this book, you've already made a great start on informing yourself about your loved one's condition. Allow the information we've included here to lead you to more, be that through online databases, specialist organisations or support groups.

What can you do?

The first thing you need to do in order to deal with this is to make sure your loved one is getting all of the necessary support, and to call in medical professionals if this has not already been done. It may feel as though you are betraying your loved one by calling in the professionals without their say-so, but know that this is the right thing to do.

Ensuring the person you love is getting the treatment they need is the only way you can make sure they are moving towards happiness and recovery. If your loved one has a history of refusing medical assistance in circumstances like this, ask her GP to explain to her why it is so vital that she gets proper help at this time, and what can happen if she refuses.

Even if she doesn't feel ready to receive outside assistance initially, she will soon reach a point where she is able to understand how important this step can be. This may be soon, or it may take a little while: everyone with postnatal depression is different, so no two cases are the same. Each case is altered by the individual's specific coping mechanisms, behaviours and needs.

The good news is that there are some tips you can try that will help sufferers in most situations and if you can keep these in mind, they'll keep you afloat while you search for other things that help.

Distinguish between person and illness

Postnatal depression often leads to a fair amount of challenging behaviour, and all you can really do is keep in mind that this isn't her, it's her condition. It isn't your loved one who is being difficult, negative or obstructive, it's the symptoms that come attached to postnatal depression. You aren't going to tell your father to just wise up and stop being difficult if he's broken his leg and needs a wheelchair.

Try to apply the same understanding to your loved one with postnatal depression.

All you can do is wait

There is no quick fix for postnatal depression – the only cure is time. Rather than looking for a cure that doesn't exist, try to offer the person you love all of the affection, security, reassurance and support you can to help them through this illness.

> There is no quick fix for postnatal depression – the only cure is time. Rather than looking for a cure that doesn't exist, try to offer the person you love all of the affection, security, reassurance and support you can to help them through this illness.

Practice being a Good Listener

As is the case with many other mental health issues, sometimes the best thing you can do for someone with postnatal depression is to listen. It doesn't matter if what they're saying doesn't make an awful lot of sense, if you don't agree or if they've told you the same thing multiple times, just give them the gift of listening. Don't nag her, offer unwanted opinions, cajole or judge, just nod and let her know she isn't alone.

Often, there will be times when your friend or family member needs more support than usual, for example if she's been put on a new medication and is experiencing new and unpleasant side effects. The most important thing you can do to help is to be understanding, consistent, non-judgemental and kind, so that your friend knows they can trust you even when they have limited control over their actions.

The difficulties your loved one is experiencing are not her fault, and she did not choose to suffer from this illness or to cause problems for her friends and family.

The difficulties your loved one is experiencing are not her fault, and she did not choose to suffer from this illness or to cause problems for her friends and family. There are some specific resources and skills that you may find useful in order to invest all of the necessary time and energy into your relationship. More than anything else, healthy communication is crucial in maintaining functional and strong relationships.

If you are simply listening, then you should focus entirely on listening to what she has to say. However, if this is a discussion, there are a few tips which can be helpful in mastering interpersonal communication:

- Take all the time you need to think about exactly what you want to say and what you are trying to communicate to your friend.

- Don't interrupt – put effort into listening.

- Try to create a shared perspective of the issue. If you can't agree on a problem, you won't be able to agree on a solution.

- Be very clear about any issues you are trying to get across, but take responsibility. Don't place responsibility for problems on your friend with postnatal depression, as it can easily lead to them becoming upset or frustrated.

- If a conversation begins to get a little heated, take some time out. It's important that you try to stay calm, as we often do and say things we regret when we're angry.

- Avoid words like 'never' or 'always', and other sweeping statements.

If you are someone who is prone to issues with anger, it may be a good idea to consider anger management courses. Your GP will be able to give you information about local resources, or you can visit the British Association of Anger Management's (BAAM) website at www.angermanage.co.uk and make use of the resources listed there. There are also a great range of self-help books about anger management available.

Make yourself available

Try to make sure to be there for her whenever she needs you. Depression can be a deeply lonely experience, and postnatal depression has the extra frightening aspect of a baby to care for. In many cases, new mothers will be anxious about being alone with their baby – not because there's a risk of harm, but because the level of close personal contact this involves can be exhausting or intense.

Of course, we understand you have a life of your own and by no means do we recommend quitting your job so that you can be waiting by the phone at all times. Simply try to make yourself a little more flexible for the time being. If things get frustrating, remember that this is only temporary.

Offering Practical Support

No matter the situation – postnatal depression or no postnatal depression – the best type of support you can give to your family and friends is the offer of strength, encouragement and love whenever it is needed. Even in families dealing with postnatal depression, this can make a vast difference and can even help your loved one deal with their illness more easily.

Try to provide as much hands-on help as you possibly can, but remember to be practical about it. The life of a carer is incredibly busy, and you'll have your own commitments to deal with at the same time. The best solution for this is to avoid trying to do it all on your own. Make sure the person you're caring for has a strong network of other carers, relatives and friends who they can contact when you aren't available.

It may be helpful to consider some of the following ideas:

- Could someone be paid to do certain duties such as gardening or cleaning?
- Could a family member make extra servings of food that can be put in the mother's freezer?

- Could you help to recognise the early warning symptoms of a low period?
- Could you keep their diary updated so they don't miss any important appointments?
- Could someone help them with household admin, such as bills?
- Are you on hand to support your friend through crises?
- Could someone collect their medication and prescriptions?
- Can you help them visit their community mental health team or GP, or accompany them to support groups?
- Could you help them to provide their GP with information about their activities and symptoms? This can help them understand the impact their medications are having, as well as assisting with talking treatments like CBT.
- Do any of your local supermarkets give the option of online shopping?
- Would anyone be available to look after the baby once per week to give the mother a break?

Some people also find it helpful to work with the person with postnatal depression to create a plan in advance in case of emergencies – things like compiling a list of useful emergency numbers and discussing what actions need to be taken in different scenarios can be useful.

Understand the importance of 'Me Time'

Offer the person suffering with postnatal depression a little time out from the usual pressures of her life. Even if this space just gives them time to have a nap, take a bath, go for a walk or pick up groceries, it'll be much appreciated and will also allow you to bond with the baby. If it's at all possible, it's a nice idea to try and make this a regular occurrence. Try putting aside the same time each week – giving this activity its own weekly timeslot will make it easier to remember to do this.

This will also give her something special that she can look forward to during the week, which can have a brilliant positive effect on the state of mind.

The Rollercoaster Ride

Postnatal depression is an illness of ups and down, so there's no point in expecting your loved one's recovery to form a neat upwards line graph. The course of their recovery will be more like a rollercoaster, or a winding country road. Some days it'll seem like she's almost back to normal and you'll start seeing the light at the end of the tunnel, and the next day things can seem worse than ever.

Try not to despair too much when this happens. This illness follows a curious course with ups and downs that'll keep you on your toes. All you can do is trust that with the right treatment and a little time and understanding, the bad days will slowly become less frequent and the person you know and love will be back.

Know that this isn't permanent

We've already advised that sufferers should routinely remind themselves that this isn't forever, but it's also a good idea for those around them to adopt the same philosophy. Keep in mind that the person you know and love isn't gone forever, she's simply going to behave a little differently for a short while. In time, everything will get back to normal and you can go back to enjoying your relationship.

Don't forget to take care of yourself

It can be easy to forget, but someone needs to take care of the carers. This is a difficult time for everyone involved. Whether the person with postnatal depression is your partner, friend, daughter or wife, it will be affecting you somehow. Please ensure that you're making an effort to keep yourself safe and happy.

Watch what you eat

Try to eat three balanced, nutritious meals each day, and drink lots and lots of water. You need to give yourself all of the necessary fuel if you want to care for your loved one to the best of your ability. If you fall ill now, that won't help anyone!

Be well

It's all very well that you've managed to guide your friend towards getting the professional help they need, but it's also important that you seek your own medical help if necessary. Caring for someone who has postnatal depression (or indeed

Keep in mind that the person you know and love isn't gone forever, she's simply going to behave a little differently for a short while. In time, everything will get back to normal and you can go back to enjoying your relationship.

any other mental health condition) can be exhausting, so don't be too proud to get help for yourself too. Even if you don't feel comfortable talking to your GP about this, you could find yourself a free counselling service.

Whatever you do, make sure there's at least one person in your life who's ready to listen to your worries and feelings. Just because your friend has this illness, it doesn't mean that your emotional needs are no longer important or significant. Be sure to confront your own issues before attempting to shoulder someone else's.

Stay Rested

Remember to take a step back from your responsibilities in life every now and again (this includes your caring duties). Allow yourself a chance to do nothing at all. Help yourself develop an awareness of your feelings and breathing, and just sit back for a while.

Dads and Depression

Research carried out by the Mental Health Foundation in 2004 has found that up to 1 in 14 fathers will suffer from postnatal depression following the birth of their child.

The men in these studies exhibited symptoms which were almost identical to those shown by new mothers. Of course, this condition is not one occurring as a result of giving birth or being pregnant. Similarly, it isn't as a result of the same hormonal, biological or psychological challenges faced by their female counterparts. There are, however, a number of explanations for why a father might experience postnatal depression.

- In cases where one partner is suffering from postnatal depression, early parenthood can become exceptionally difficult for a new father.

- First time fathers are often vulnerable as they can find it more difficult to deal with changes to their usual sleep patterns and routines. They also often experience extreme pressure and anxiety levels as a result of becoming the sole breadwinner of the household.

- It's common to experience depression as a result of a sudden change in the dynamics of your relationship.

- Men who have a history of depression and mental illnesses are very likely to experience depression following their child's birth.

- Men who become fathers later in life are more prone to depression, for the same reasons as first-time fathers.

What help is available for new fathers?

The best way to deal with your new status as a father is to implement a rule of openness and honesty. If you find yourself feeling lost, anxious or depressed, don't let your pride get in the way of finding help before you reach crisis point. Make yourself talk about your feeling with your close friends, GP, family or partner. It's common for men to find themselves functioning under the misguided societal idea that all they need to do is 'man up' and get on with it. Don't let this be you.

The best thing you can do in your situation is to look for the help that you need, and be honest about how you are feeling. This might feel like a step that you aren't ready to take, and that's ok. Here are a few tips to make your search for improved mental health go that little bit more smoothly.

- Begin by understanding that there are no quick fixes or shortcuts when it comes to dealing with postnatal depression. This isn't some minor issue you can just get over, but it is something you can work through over time. In time you will reach the other end of your journey as an emotionally stronger and better informed person.

- Even if it feels like nobody else is trying to help, treat your recovery as a team effort. As it stands, the healthcare system is very enthusiastic about supporting new mothers through all of their worries and problems. However, they're rarely quite so concerned about the wellbeing of the father. Always remember that parenting is generally done through a team strategy, and that your position on that team is just as important as that of the mother.

- Don't wait for someone to ask before opening up. Fathers are very often forgotten during early parenthood, so try your best not to become the next in a long line of invisible sufferers. Make yourself heard. Tell people – your pals, your family, your partner – all about what you're going through. Just opening up a little bit can relieve some stress and help you feel more human.

- Just talking to a friend or family member is a massive step towards recovery, but please don't leave your GP out of the equation. Your doctor is still the best person to talk to in order to make a healthy, steady recovery. They'll also have some helpful advice and support which can improve your life and that of your family.

- Try and find local societies and support groups that meet in your area. It's unlikely you'll be able to find one specifically aimed at men with postnatal depression, but there should still be a group that you can go to to let your feelings out a little.

- Remind yourself (and, if necessary, those around you) that being the father doesn't simply mean being 'the provider,' and that your mental and physical health are just as important to the wellbeing of your family. Destroy the notion that the father is simply a spare part, you are absolutely vital.

- Don't let yourself be fooled into believing that postnatal depression is a condition that only affects women. It takes two people to create a new human being, so it is a process that impacts both of you. Suffering from postnatal depression does not reflect negatively on your masculinity.

What have we learned?

It's vital that we keep in mind mothers aren't the only people who need looked after when it comes to postnatal depression. Carers are often forgotten about in this respect. Whether you're a grandparent, friend or father, there's plenty of help available if you know where to look. Try to make sure you're fully informed about postnatal depression, and be open and honest about your experiences.

New fathers can also suffer from postnatal depression. Try to identify whether you are at risk, and learn the steps you can take to try and make things easier for you. Always remember that all the best carers know to look after themselves as well. As with any other mental health condition, the symptoms of postnatal depression vary from person to person, but there are a few important rules that apply to most situations.

Try to view the recovery process as a long road you both need to walk down. As with any other road, this one will reach its destination and come to an end. Try to create a sense of flexibility, security, comfort and space for your loved one. Become the best carer you can be by taking all of the steps necessary to take proper care of yourself.

10

Doing it all over again

You'd be forgiven for thinking that once you've had one child, you are a mother and any other babies will just be the same again. You know what to expect, you've done it before. But think again. Every baby will be different, and being a mother is an experience that will just keep changing. Sadly, this means there's every chance you can suffer from postnatal depression more than once.

Postnatal depression: The second time around

In fact, it's actually far more likely for you to struggle with postnatal depression the second time you give birth. Research suggests that the incidence for this could be anywhere up to 60%, and nobody has figured out exactly why this is the case. It seems as though postnatal depression is something you will or won't be 'prone' to. Patterns can be spotted down through families, so it makes sense that if you've already dealt with the condition once, you can easily get it again.

This may sound completely unfair on those who've already gone through this once, but it's also bad for people for whom their second born brings the first experience of postnatal depression. You think you've done it all once, that you're a veteran and that there's nothing they can throw at you that you haven't defeated once before, and then postnatal depression knocks you off your feet right out of the blue.

And just like every baby being different, every case of postnatal illness is unique. So just how is one supposed to deal with this alongside your new baby and older children?

Welcome to Round Two

Babies are incredibly needy and will take up vast amounts of your time. Having two babies to look after (however old your first child is by now) is going to be twice as difficult. If you somehow managed to have 'me time' with your first child, don't fall into the trap of expecting the second to be as accommodating.

When you had your first child, the advice was to sleep when the baby slept to make up for all those sleepless nights, but it's highly unlikely that your child will be interested in this plan when their baby sibling comes into the world. Chances are, your older kid will be just as excited as you are about the baby being asleep, because it means they finally have you to themselves. And who are you to deny them time with their parents?

Suddenly your baby is awake again and needs fed, and a full nap time has gone by without a moment's rest for you.

The extra exhaustion and busyness that comes with caring for two children of different ages can easily trigger a new bout of depression. The relationship between a parent and their child is often the most intense feeling of love in the human experience. But when the number of children doubles, it's easy to see how parents can begin to wonder if they have the energy to feel this amount of love for two children at once.

Will my relationship with my firstborn suffer?

Once they've brought more new life into the world, it's common for a mother to experience a sense of loss (ironic, right?). This is because they begin to lament the loss of time that they once spent with their older child or children. It's also common to experience a strong feeling of guilt over spending less time with your other children, which only becomes more difficult to deal with when combined with postnatal depression.

Sibling rivalries

When new babies arrive, they have a massive impact on the family dynamic and it's easy for their older siblings to feel forgotten. Suddenly, all of the attention they were used to receiving has been redirected towards this new infant, and they may begin to act out in order to regain some of this attention. They begin to feel as though it's something they need to earn, rather than something they'll be given for simply existing.

Even if none of this happens and your older children are enthusiastic, unaffected and self-assured, your own sense of guilt can easily be enough to make you feel as though you are not doing everything a good parent needs to do.

Is it worth going through it all again?

You're going to hear over and over again that in time, your body makes you forget all of the exhaustion, the physical discomforts and the dramas of childbirth. This, alas, is not the case: most mothers will remember all to clearly all of this horror as soon as their next due date begins to loom. The second or third time you give birth, you'll not only be dealing with your current experiences but will be layering these on to your massive stack of negative memories.

This will only serve to increase the anxiety you'll need to deal with: Will you manage? Will the birth be easier or more difficult? These worries can easily spin out of control long before your new baby comes into the world. If you're predisposed to suffering from postnatal depression, this can cause a great amount of distress.

While every life that comes into the world is special in its own way, the second baby you give birth to can sometimes feel a little less special if you're already having a hard time with your feelings. This can make things very hard, as can the massive decrease in time you can dedicate to self-care and self-love.

And once you're a mum, you're expected to be a professional parent who can leap back into action the second the cord is cut. In fact, even the hospital will expect you to have vacated your bed within 48 hours so they can bring in the next mum-to-be.

What can you do about it?

When it comes to confronting postnatal depression the second time, your best plan of action is to scrap the defensive and go on the offensive. This sounds like a massive mountain to climb, but it's entirely possible. Use careful planning and hope to guide you through.

Know what might be coming

One of the major advantages you'll have for your second child is that you'll know all about some of the things you can expect to experience. If you've already have postnatal depression, you already know which warning signs to look out for and what is and isn't 'normal' for you. All of your friends and family will have a better understanding of what they can do to help, too.

Look after yourself

Take care to support yourself properly during pregnancy and early motherhood. This includes eating a healthy, balanced diet and getting help with your other children when you need it. If your children are old enough to go to school, try asking someone else to take on some of their school runs, or to take them to their extra-curricular activities.

Remember that getting the rest you need isn't a luxury, it's an essential if you wish to be happy and healthy. Being properly rested also means you'll have more energy to give your older children the attention they need.

Ahead of your due date, make sure that you have a strong support network in place.

Hope for the best

Know that there's every chance this pregnancy will be just as difficult as the last, but don't let that keep you from staying positive. Remind yourself that the worst won't necessarily happen, and feel comfortable and safe in the knowledge that if lightning does strike again, you know how to deal with it.

What medical help is available?

If you're worried about going through postnatal depression again, try talking to your doctor as there is a great range of medical help they can offer.

Preventative antidepressants

Some doctors will be more than happy to offer you a course of antidepressants to take over the final weeks of your pregnancy if they feel you are vulnerable to postnatal depression. However, there are certain risks that come with taking medication at this point, and it's important that you discuss these in detail before deciding whether you'd rather take them now or wait until after the birth to begin treatment.

Importantly, any drugs you are offered should be carefully chosen to minimise any potential risks to your unborn child.

Hormone Replacement Therapy (HRT)

This more controversial means of treating recurring postnatal depression was pioneered by Dr Katharina Dalton, who advocated working against the potential return of postnatal depression by a hormonal approach. While some experts believe that this HRT should be beneficial to new mothers, some women have reported that the treatment has only served to worsen their health.

This method was to include the use of progesterone replacement therapies to treat the mother. The idea was that the therapy would counteract the major reduction of this hormone in the mother's system following childbirth. This is a drop which some experts suggest can be extremely detrimental to the mental health of new mothers in their most vulnerable stages.

Pregnancy counselling

Many worried mothers find talking treatments and other forms of psychological support to be incredibly effective during their pregnancy. These treatments might involve discussing any concerns you have about giving birth (which can be especially helpful following a traumatic previous birth), CBT (cognitive behavioural therapy) or straightforward counselling. CBT especially is a highly effective method which involves learning techniques which allow you to change destructive thought patterns into more positive, helpful ones.

Older Children

Trying to deal with postnatal depression while caring for both new babies and their siblings can be very tricky. Don't panic, though! If you keep pushing through, you can do this.

Help them understand what's happening

Make sure that you explain the changes you might experience to your older children, and help them understand that any new or unusual behaviour is just because you're getting used to looking after their new baby brother or sister. This will reassure the child and help them to relate to you, as that's exactly what they're trying to do at the moment too.

Make nap time a team activity

Sharing rest times with your older children, such as relaxing together while the baby is sleeping, can help them feel more responsible, grown up and closer to you. Create a miniature home cinema by just watching a DVD with popcorn and snuggles. Try making a little pillow fort, or gathering some books that you can read together.

Getting the big brothers and sisters involved with rest times can help you to really take the time to enjoy them, and the new novelty of spending time with a child who is less likely to cry, teethe or need their nappy changed. Make sure you keep this as a restful time, though: physical activities can be saved for afternoons where you have someone else looking after the baby.

Give them responsibilities

Often, your older children will be only too excited to help with their new baby sibling. Finding and fetching the supplies you need gives them attention and purpose, and means you'll have more time to spend with them when the work is done.

Accept challenging behaviour

If you want to keep the peace in your house, it may be necessary to ignore some of your older children's bad behaviour. Even if it's something you'd usually scold them for, unless it's an actively dangerous action, it can be easier to simply turn a blind eye. If your child is feeling ignored or forgotten, drawing attention to a negative action might simply show them that acting out is an effective way to get noticed.

What have we learned?

One of the most important tools when coping with postnatal depression for the second time is foresight. Better planning allows for better prevention. Your primary defence against postnatal depression is all of the little, simple measures you can put in place in advance. Make sure you're getting all of the rest you need and eating a healthy, balanced diet.

As your due date grows nearer, make sure you have a safe and strong support system made up of relatives and friends. These people will be more than happy to help you with errands, older siblings and chores. Find different ways of getting your older children involved in the care of their new baby brother or sister, and make sure they're still getting all of the affection, love and cuddles they need.

Just like you'd make a birth plan or a fitness plan, try to make a wellbeing plan for yourself. Think about all the ways you'd like to work through your postnatal depression differently this time. Your doctor and other healthcare providers will also have lots of help to offer you. If your family doctor believes it's a good idea, try talking about the option of taking antidepressants during the last few weeks of your pregnancy. Talking therapies and HRT are also available.

The second time you give birth, you are highly likely to suffer from postnatal depression. This may well come down to any number of different mental, lifestyle or physical factors. Because nobody has worked out the exact cause of postnatal depression, your best bet is to confront the condition in every way possible. If you put plenty of safety measures in place, you'll be better off whether you experience this second bout of depression or not. If you do experience postnatal depression, you'll be well prepared to deal with it better the second time.

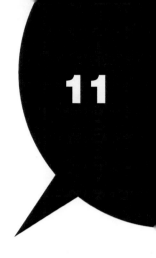

11

Which Medications Can Help?

One common and understandable response to the suggestion of taking medication is anxiety about not wanting to fill yourself with chemicals. There are loads of myths floating around about antidepressants that make them seem very intimidating and unhealthy. Combine these with some common-garden misjudgement, ignorance and a good dose of media horror stories and you get the idea that pharmaceuticals should only be used as a last resort, if at all.

While understandable, these objections are completely unfounded: if you were suffering from a condition like arthritis, diabetes or kidney disease, nobody would have a problem with you taking the necessary medications to improve your symptoms. It's simply the stigma, society's belief that requiring antidepressants is a sign of inadequacy or weakness, or that taking them will cause you to turn to illegal drugs, that is standing between you and recovery.

With proper consideration, choice and understanding, antidepressants can be a real life-saver if your postnatal depression becomes overwhelming. Sadly, medication isn't a magic spell that will instantly cure you of postnatal depression. It can take weeks, even months, of working with your doctor or psychiatrist to perfect your dosage. It's a good idea to pursue treatment as soon after the development of your symptoms as possible, so that you can work with your doctor to get the best treatment you can, as soon as you can.

If you find yourself on a medication or dosage you aren't happy with, keep in mind that coming off the medication very suddenly can make you very ill. Nobody will force you to stay on a medication you don't want to be taking, but it's important that you discuss with your doctor first so that you know the safest, most effective way of ending that particular form of treatment.

Why should I opt for antidepressants?

Make the choice to stop seeing taking the medication you need as a sign of weakness, and understand that it's a sign of strength. Taking antidepressants can be something which will better your life along with those of your baby and other family members.

This isn't to be seen as giving up or giving in. As with any other drugs, choosing antidepressants needs to be a conscious and informed decision.

Importantly, antidepressants do not alter your mind. They alter the chemicals in your brain so that they reach the same levels as everyone else's. You aren't going to turn into a different person – you'll just be you, but in a better mood.

Medication for Depression

There are lots of personality types out there, and each one is determined by the chemical make-up of the brain. Because chemical make-ups vary so much from person to person, and because antidepressants work by acting on these chemicals, there are a variety of different antidepressants in existence.

This is why an antidepressant which is prescribed to one patient might not be an option for another patient, or simply won't work. A GP needs to consider carefully which type of medication suits each of their patients the best, and to revise these choices depending on the side effects the patient experiences.

Depression is believed to stem from a chemical imbalance in the brain, which can be addressed by medication. Alterations are made by changing the levels of different neurotransmitters – chemicals which conduct electrical impulses between neurons – in the brain. It is these chemicals that regulate or control a number of your bodily functions, including your mood. Experts believe that depression is caused by a lack of the neurotransmitters serotonin and noradrenaline.

Remember that every drug has potential side effects, which are outlined in detail by their manufacturers. Because everyone is different, there's a chance you'll experience these side effects severely, mildly or not at all. If you do experience side effects which are interfering with your daily life, be sure to inform your GP so they can review your medication or dosage.

Your antidepressants should take somewhere between 2 and 8 weeks to start working, so you should continue to take them even if they don't appear to be having an effect initially. In some cases, individuals are able to come off their antidepressants as soon as their depression appears to have ended, but in others you'll be expected to stay on the medication for a number of months. It all depends on how you have reacted to antidepressants in the past. Either way, you should not stop taking antidepressants suddenly: dosage should be gradually reduced over a number of weeks.

The following are some of the most commonly used antidepressants at present.

Tricyclic Antidepressants (TCAs)

- Allegron (nortriptyline)
- Prothiaden (dothiepin)
- Surmontil (trimipramine)
- Imipramine
- Amitriptyline
- Anafranil SR (clomipramine)
- Lomont (lofepramine)
- Sinepin (doxepin)
- Anafranil (clomipramine)

The oldest type of antidepressant, tricyclics are less specifically targeted than their newer counterparts and often have more side-effects as a result. Aside from this, though, they work on a similar principle to the other drugs you might be prescribed. Tricyclics have a tendency towards making people feel sleepy and drowsy, especially in the cases of dothiepin and amitriptyline.

Although this can be beneficial to those who are restless or anxious, it's not so good if you're trying to care for an infant. Tricyclic antidepressants like lofepramine and imipramine have less of a sedative effect than others. TCAs can bring with them a variety of other side effects which may include difficulty in urinating, dry mouth, weight gain, blurred vision and constipation.

It is strongly advised that those who suffer from heart disease should not be prescribed tricyclic antidepressants. Your doctor is only likely to prescribe these if other antidepressants have been unsuccessful. Drugs such as venlafaxine work in a similar way to TCAs, but without producing these side effects.

SNRI antidepressants

SNRIs were developed after SSRIs, and are seen as another step up from them. Although the two types work on the same principle, SNRIs are also designed to work on the chemical noradrenalin in your brain. These drugs may be prescribed if SSRIs have been unsuccessful.

Monoamine oxidase inhibitors (MAOIs)

- Isocarboxazid
- Tranylcypromine
- Manerix (moclobemide)
- Nardil (phenelzine)

This is a category of drugs which are very rarely prescribed, as their chemistry means they can react badly with other substances and medications, even including over-the-counter cold and flu medicines. In some cases, these drugs can even cause serious reactions with everyday food items.

In the unlikely event that you are prescribed one of these drugs, you will need to be placed on a very specific diet and under careful supervision. Rather than interacting with the your brain chemicals like other antidepressants, MAOIs work by altering the enzymes that work on the chemicals.

A newer type of MAOI, moclobemide is more likely to be prescribed than other MAOIs. This drug appears to cause fewer adverse effects than other similar medications, but it's still advised that those taking this medication exercise great caution around certain medicines and foods.

Selective Serotonin Reuptake Inhibitors (SSRIs)

These include:

- Cipralex (escitalopram)

- Lustral (sertraline)

- Cipramil (citalopram)

- Faverin (fluvoxamine)

- Seroxat (paroxetine)

- Prozac (fluoxetine)

Of the SSRIs listed above, fluoxetine is generally used the least often as it stays in the body for a long time after treatment has ended. SSRIs were developed more recently than MAOIs (monoamine oxidase inhibitors) and tricyclics, and have all but replaced them in most cases. They work by specifically targeting the happy hormone, serotonin, and stopping it from being broken down. This means your serotonin levels will be increased, reducing your depressive feelings and improving your mood.

Because SSRIs are more targeted in their actions, they tend to cause fewer side effects than tricyclics. However, they do still carry potential side effects including anxiousness, reduced sexual function and insomnia. While all antidepressants have been found to be linked with sexual difficulties like impotence, this issue seems to occur most frequently with SSRIs.

Other side effects can include vomiting, constipation, diarrhoea and nausea. As they have far fewer sedative effects than older types of antidepressant, SSRIs are more suitable for people who feel their depression slows them down, and especially those with heart problems.

As with other antidepressants, SSRIs do not raise your mood straight away. They generally take somewhere between two and four weeks to produce any noticeable effects, and any improvements will be gradual. Even after four weeks have passed, it's unlikely you will have experienced their full effects. It's important to just be patient and give your medication time to work.

Can I take antidepressants if I'm pregnant or breastfeeding?

The unavoidable fact of the matter is that if you take antidepressants while pregnant or breastfeeding, they will reach your baby. This means that certain antidepressants which could potentially affect your baby's health will be off the table, but there are plenty of other options. Many antidepressants will only reach your baby in negligible amounts, and will easily leave the baby's system without causing damage.

Even when taking higher dosages of antidepressants, many women choose to breastfeed.

Although it is not yet known what the exact long-term effects of this will be on the babies, there have yet to be any real signs or concerns which would cause alarm. This is a case where you just have to think in pros and cons. Would leaving your depression untreated have worse consequences for the future happiness and health of your family than risking treatment?

Try also looking into other types of treatment which would allow you to reduce your dosage of medication (or stop taking it altogether) without putting your own health and wellbeing at risk. Don't consider the medication you need to no longer be an option as a result of breastfeeding or pregnancy. Educate yourself, and make informed decisions based on all of the options you have.

Whatever you choose, your health visitor and GP will be there to support you and help you with your decisions.

Coming off your antidepressants

Don't make the mistake of thinking you're cured and stopping your medication as soon as your antidepressants stop to work. You can't just instantly go back to normal. Most doctors will ask you to take your medication for at least six months. This will help reduce the likelihood of the condition recurring in the future, and give you some time for recovery.

Importantly, before you begin to stop your tablets, you need talk to your GP about how to go about it. Withdrawing very suddenly can be dangerous. Understand that although antidepressants aren't addictive, you can still experience withdrawal symptoms if you stop taking them. Most experts will suggest that you gradually reduce your dosage over a number of months to make the process gentler.

Always follow your GP's advice

Make sure you have all the information about side effects, etc. This will help you to feel more in control of your situation. However, be careful not to over-research or convince yourself into experiencing unnecessary symptoms. It's vital that you have the support of your friends, family or partner at this time. They need to know what you're doing so that they know what to expect.

Once you've settled on coming of your medication, make sure you do this at a time when your life feels under control and settled. For example, it's probably best not to start while you're preparing for a holiday or in the run-up to Christmas.

Dos and Don'ts

If you carefully follow all of the tips and guidelines you're given, your experience of antidepressants should go smoothly.

Do

- Source as much information as you can on different antidepressants and how each one works. Discuss each of your options in detail with your GP.

- Make sure you keep your tablets somewhere safe and out of reach, as they can do real damage if they're taken by the wrong person or in the wrong dosage. This is especially important if there are children in your house.

- Give your tablets plenty of time to get to work. Most antidepressants will take around two to four weeks to begin working properly. Even if you begin to feel better soon after beginning your treatment, it's best to remain on your medication for at least six months.

- Tell your GP if you begin to experience any side effects while on antidepressants. They may recommend that you wait until your mood improves before changing anything, or they may decide to change your dosage or medication.

- Find out if there are any other substances you'll need to avoid. In some cases, St John's wort or alcohol can have severe effects when combined with antidepressants.

- Meet with your GP on a regular basis for review and check-ups. Talk to them about important medical tests like blood pressure checks, as well as about how you are feeling.

- Try treating your depression with a combination of treatments, like combining your medication with something like counselling, relaxation or cognitive behavioural therapy. Depression is usually less straightforward than a solitary chemical imbalance, and we're yet to work out exactly what causes it. It's best to treat the condition by all means possible.

- Get yourself into a healthy routine by taking your medication around the same time each day. Make your treatment part of your everyday life. Certain medications will involve taking only one tablet each day, while others will require two. If this is the case, try taking one in the morning and one at night.

Don't

- Assume 'natural' or 'herbal' substances are automatically safe for you to take. These can still react with your medication.

- Expect antidepressants to be a magical cure that will get rid of your depression forever. They can help to relieve your symptoms, but there may also be environmental causes which you'll need to deal with in different ways.

- Get disheartened if the first antidepressant you try doesn't work for you. Not all medications work for everyone. There will be a medication out there that works for you.

- Change your own dosage based on how you're feeling. Your doses should be constant, regular and even. You should never change your prescription details without talking to your psychiatrist or GP first.

What have we learned?

Don't let social stigma stop you from considering antidepressants. These medications have been studied, developed and redeveloped over decades to make them as safe and effective as possible, and there's something out there that will suit everyone. Do your homework, so that you and your GP can work together to find the medication that works best for you.

It can also be beneficial to research other treatments you can try alongside medication, such as talking therapies. Don't base your decisions on any myths or prejudices, especially when it comes to something as important as your mental health. Society has a lot of misconceptions about antidepressants, and to miss out on treatment that could greatly improve your quality of life because of these would be an unfortunate and sad mistake.

12

Other Options for Treatment

There are a great number of options you can try in the treatment of your postnatal depression. Some of these are considered to be fairly alternative and some are downright controversial, but all of them are worth researching.

A note to the reader

Alternative treatments are often viewed to be 'better' or 'healthier' simply because they are 'natural'. Please keep in mind that a great number of traditional drugs and medications are made from natural substances, and are made available by prescription because it's possible to react dangerously or overdose if these substances are taken without due care.

Something being 'natural' or 'herbal' doesn't necessarily make it good for you, and certainly doesn't mean that you should take it freely without proper medical information. Similarly, just because you require a prescription to access certain traditional medicines doesn't make them 'unnatural' or 'unhealthy'. If you do choose to try alternative treatments, please talk to your GP first so they can explain how to go about this safely.

St John's wort

The use of St John's wort as a 'natural' alternative to traditional antidepressants has been recommended for years, and with great foundation. This substance acts as the perfect reminder that herbal alternatives should be treated with great care. Some of the substances derived from plants have been used to make the most toxic poisons we have. Others are used in the medications that keep us healthy. For example, foxglove (digitalis) is used in heart medicines.

St John's wort is no exception to the rule of requiring great care. Many people have found it to be an impressive and effective treatment for mild and moderate depression, although some have experienced side effects similar to those found with traditional antidepressants.

Also known as hypericum, St John's wort is a plant which has small, yellow flowers. It's been used to treat a variety of condition for hundreds of years. You can find it in most supermarkets and healthfood stores, often in the form of capsules or tablets.

Importantly, there's no hard evidence that this product works as a treatment for depression. We must simply rely on the outcomes described by those who have taken the drug. Based on these testimonies, it's believed that St John's wort works by impacting the balance of brain chemicals like noradrenalin and serotonin. This would mean it works in a similar way to SSRI antidepressants.

There are also even more similarities in the gradual improvement the plant seems to cause in the mood, as well as the waiting time of two to four weeks for the drug's full effects. The main benefit of taking St John's wort is that its side effects appear to be less severe than those of prescribed antidepressants, which is sometimes considered to make the drug well worth the lack of research.

Do take care, though: St John's wort can have a negative impact on the effectiveness of any other antidepressants, blood-thinning or contraceptive medications you are taking. This means the plant should only be taken after professional consultation, and shouldn't be taken at all if you're pregnant or breastfeeding.

Hormone Replacement Therapy (HRT)

It makes sense: After you give birth, you experience massive changes in your levels of oestrogen along with a whopping 120% drop in your levels of progesterone. Knowing that these hormones have an effect on your mental, emotional and physical state, it's not shocking that when there are drastic changes in their levels (for example during pregnancy, menopause, childbirth or menstruation), it can impact your mental and physical health dramatically.

Research has pointed on a number of different occasions to the possibility of hormonal treatments being an effective treatment for the resulting conditions, including postnatal depression.

What does the treatment entail?

The original idea behind hormone replacement therapy is that the symptoms of postnatal depression could be cancelled out by a series of injections and pessaries immediately after giving birth. Some people believe that this is safe as the hormone progesterone should be in the body naturally and therefore would pose little to no risk to her health or that of her baby.

Some doctors dispute the effectiveness of HRT when used to treat postnatal depression, and it's still considered to be a controversial treatment so you may want to do some research into it before making any decisions. To help your search, here are just a few interesting websites with information on the treatment:

- Progesterone Link is a website which features information about progesterone therapy. (www.progesteronelink.com)

- NaProTECHNOLOGY (Natural Procreative Technology) is a new women's health science which focuses on women's gynecological and reproductive health. Their website contains a very good page discussing postnatal depression and the work of Dr Dalton. (www.naprotechnology.com)

- The Natural-Progesterone-Advisory-Network is a Women's Hormonal Health. Community advocating proper information on safe and effective use and dosage guidelines for bioidentical progesterone. (www.natural-progesterone-advisory-network.com)

While the information on these websites may come in handy, don't forget that these are commercial sites, and it's important to search for separate, unbiased information where possible.

Nutritional therapy

As we have said over and over again throughout this book: A healthy, balanced diet is vital when recovering from postnatal depression or any other illness. Research has been carried out into how diet can provide answers for more effective postnatal depression treatment. One idea propelling this research is that while in the womb, a foetus quite literally drains the nutrients from the mother's system.

Experts have suggested that deficiencies in certain nutrients could be a major contributing factor to postnatal depression. A lot of popular theories are circulating as a result that new mothers should increase their intake of nutrients like vitamin B, omega-3 fatty acids, magnesium and zinc. While no two bodies are the same and nutritional deficiencies will impact everyone differently, it makes sense to try taking some supplements and see if you feel any better.

If you're unsure where to begin, you could try making an appointment with a dietitian, especially one who specialises in postnatal care.

Complementary therapies

Some approaches won't work as treatment for postnatal depression in their own right, but can be helpful when used to complement other forms of treatment. These complementary therapies work by managing postnatal depression on a wider front.

Some mothers find some of these treatments extremely helpful, while finding other treatments to be no help at all. As with everything, they vary from person to person.

Rather than simply treating a narrow range of issues and symptoms by chemical means, complementary therapies aim to help your emotional, spiritual and physical health recover. They come as an opportunity to look around and find a treatment that sounds good to you.

- The ancient Chinese practice of acupuncture involves the insertion of metallic needles at specific points in the skin. It is believed that in doing this, the body's energy pathways are reopened and relieved.

- Hypnotherapy aims to promote healthy thought patterns and healing by accessing the deeper levels of the mind.

- Homeopathy claims to induce the human mind and body's natural healing abilities using negligible amounts of natural plant extracts.

- Osteopathy aims to treat health conditions by targeting the muscles and joints throughout the body.

- Reflexology works on the idea that your feet contain all of the important nerve endings in your body, and that medical conditions can therefore be treated by manipulating the soles of the feet.

- Originally a popular treatment for seasonal affective disorder (SAD), light therapy aims to promote a sense of wellbeing and rebalance hormones through the use of concentrated light rays.

- Aromatherapy is believed to improve your wellbeing, create feelings of renewal and relaxation, and deeply affect your emotions through the use of essential oils and massage.

Some of these ideas may seem a little out there but if you find that one of them improves your condition, it doesn't really matter what other people think of it. The important thing to consider here is how the treatment makes you feel, and how effective it is. Just keep in mind that everyone is different, and so not every method will help every patient. You are free to explore your options and choose a treatment that works for you.

Intensive relaxation techniques

Life can be stressful enough when you're just trying to look after yourself, let alone caring for a new infant. It can be difficult to get your thoughts to slow down a little. Some people suffering from postnatal depression experience a sense of mania or hyperactivity, while others find it simply impossible to sleep. It's important that you allow yourself to relax your body and mind, and this can require special techniques at such a busy time.

If at all possible, you should try to incorporate relaxation into your everyday life, though this can be tough at the best of times. Try to build a relaxation section into your structured recovery plan to make sure you allow yourself this time. A little time dedicated to relaxing can do a world of good, improving your sense of wellbeing, reducing your anxiety and stress levels and decreasing your breathing rates and blood pressure.

Some approaches you may find helpful include yoga, meditation, deep breathing exercises, Pilates and massage. It's important that you learn to do these things properly, and you can do this by joining a class or booking an appointment with a practitioner in one of these areas. These classes and appointments also mean you have made a commitment to carry out these activities for yourself.

What have we learned?

Everyone experiences conditions like postnatal depression differently, so it's important that you find the treatments that suit your specific case. If you feel it may be helpful, you can try methods which are less conventional than those on offer from your GP. Before undertaking such treatments, you should talk to your GP to make sure they're safe to combine with any medication or treatments you're already receiving.

Don't fall into the trap of believing that just because something is 'herbal,' it don't pose any health risks or issues. All of the most powerful substances we have – both medicines and poisons – are 'natural'. All treatments should be considered with full information and care. Many of these treatments are yet to be properly explored by science, but what's important is whether they help you feel better or not.

13

Talking Therapies

f you do just one thing today to help yourself feel better, you should try talking. There are three main areas when it comes to treating postnatal depression. Medication, which we discussed in Chapter Eleven (Which Medications Can Help?), is one. No matter what other treatment you undergo, it is vital that you remember to take any medication you are prescribed every day in order to manage your symptoms effectively.

Self care, which we discussed in Chapter Seven: How to Take Proper Care of Yourself, is also an important step in taking control over your condition. However, probably the most important part of your treatment for postnatal depression is the talking therapies, which we will discuss in this chapter. Talk to your relatives, your GP or your friends to get your journey to recovery on the road.

As the name would suggest, talking therapies involve you talking to a professional about any issues you have, either individually or as part of a group. Never underestimate the potential a simple conversation can have in helping you feel better. A great amount of research has found that a combination of talking therapies and medication is significantly more effective than medication on its own.

Talking therapies are available to you, and ready to use alongside medicinal treatments, alternative therapies or on their own. This means that it's important for you to have a good understanding of the different approaches and their effects, as well as how long they take to be effective and whether you need to access them through the NHS or through private healthcare.

Talking to friends and family

A problem shared is a problem halved, and this is the case even for serious conditions like postnatal depression. The emotional stress you are experiencing is massive, but it won't seem like such an unmanageable burden if you share it with people you trust in a comfortable setting. By sharing your worries and issues, you are not only lightening the burden you have to carry, but enhancing your relationship with the person you are talking to.

A problem shared is a problem halved, and this is the case even for serious conditions like postnatal depression.

Talking about your worries and fears will allow you to create trust, a bond which will strengthen your already valuable relationships. Getting another person involved also opens your situation to options and thoughts with an outsider's perspective. Maybe the person you talk to has even gone through postnatal depression or something similar before you, and will have specific insight which will help you plan your recovery.

It's important that we work to destroy the existing stigma around emotional difficulties, and we can do this by talking openly. Taboos will begin to disappear the second we start talking about our hidden experiences, and we can even gain new love and respect from those with whom we choose to share. Talking about our problems is a sign that we are strong.

Counselling

A counsellor sees a client in a private and confidential setting to explore a difficulty the client is having, distress they may be experiencing or perhaps their dissatisfaction with life, or loss of direction and purpose.

This is the BACP*'s description of counselling, which we find one step up from the casual talking therapy you can get by simply talking to your partner or family. This is the most straightforward type of formal talking therapy, and the talking treatment that's most widely available in the UK. *British Association for Counselling and Psychotherapy (www.bacp.co.uk)

Counselling works by focusing on you and your needs, so your therapist will do everything in their power to make sure you feel safe during your sessions together. In this treatment, your counsellor listens carefully to what you have to say in order to get an idea of your life and the issues you are struggling with from your own perspective.

This is an opportunity to say what you need to say, and know that it'll be listened to with understanding and without judgement, and that it will not go beyond you and your therapist. A big part of a counsellor's job is being empathetic towards their clients. Your therapist will be able to listen to your concerns impartiality, escaping the bias that comes with talking to close friends and family.

The aim is to help you see your difficulties from a different perspective (this is known as reframing), while providing an unbiased, non-judgemental and safe space for you to talk about the things that are bothering you. This should mean you will be more comfortable when discussing your ideas, feelings and experiences. Many people also find counselling helpful when it comes to venting repressed feelings like fear, embarrassment, grief or anger – feelings which you might not be comfortable discussing with other people in your life.

If you are finding it impossible to see any way out of your depression, your counsellor's job is to show you the paths you have. They won't be able to tell you which way you need to go, but they'll make sure you have the information you need to make informed decisions. There are a number of different types of counselling, including psychodynamic, behavioural, cognitive or humanistic (more information on this is available on the BACP website). The type your counsellor provides will depend on their theoretical perspective.

If you are referred to a counsellor by your GP, you will be offered anywhere up to six sessions. However, if you choose to see a counsellor privately, this timeframe will be much more flexible and you will be able to decide after a number of sessions whether you want or need more.

Many people also find counselling helpful when it comes to venting repressed feelings like fear, embarrassment, grief or anger – feelings which you might not be comfortable discussing with other people in your life.

Cognitive behavioural therapy

CBT therapists would argue that the way in which you think about things can have a massive impact on the way you feel, on your mood and emotions. This then goes on to affect your behaviour. Cognitive behavioural therapy (CBT) works on the basis that human beings are weighed down by the routines and prejudices which control the way they view everything that goes on around them.

Our brains are wired to react to the things we see and feel according to the ideas we already have programmed in our heads. The goal of CBT is to interrupt this process by deconstructing your thought patterns and reconstructing them in more productive, helpful and appropriate ways. The way you react to experiences will be far more positive and calm when thought through properly.

This can be done by considering the strong link that exists between thoughts and actions. In order for you to benefit fully from CBT, you'll need to commit to making it a part of your life for a number of months. It will be worth it, though, as the skills you learn can help you for the rest of your life.

What happens in CBT sessions?

As a general rule, you and your CBT therapist will meet between 5 and 20 times, on a weekly or fortnightly basis. Sessions usually last between 30 and 60 minutes. In the first couple of sessions, the therapist will explain exactly what this sort of treatment will entail, and make sure you are comfortable continuing. They'll also ask questions to find out more about your background and everyday life.

While the focus of this therapy will be on the here and now, it can be helpful to talk about the past in order to work out how it might be affecting you today. From there, treatment will involve the following factors:

- Deciding what issues you want help with in the short, medium and long term. You and your therapist will generally also start each session by discussing what you want to talk about that day.

- Doing your homework. Some therapists give homework, usually asking you to practice methods you have discussed in your everyday life.

- Breaking problems down into their separate parts. To help with this, you might be asked to begin keeping a diary so that you can keep a record of your thought patterns, feelings and actions.

- Working out how to alter unrealistic thought processes and actions.

- Looking at your thought patterns, emotions and actions. Together, you can decide which responses were helpful or unhelpful, realistic or unrealistic. You can then figure out how these behaviours affect you and those around you.

How CBT can help regulate your mood

Although they can feel very much internal, your emotions are generally influenced by a combination of external factors – such as the nature of your work – and internal ones like self-critical or otherwise negative thoughts. It is your CBT therapist's job to help you understand how these factors work together to impact your mood. However, it's also important to remember that a certain amount of variation in your mood is entirely normal and healthy.

CBT teaches that mood doesn't need to be a problem, that it's the way in which we think about the mood that turns it into a problem. Moods themselves only become a problem when they lead to strange or harmful behaviours. Keep in mind that everyone's moods change from time to time. It is only when they begin to interfere with your life or the lives of those around you that you should begin to worry.

Psychotherapy

People have been intrigued by psychotherapy for years. The practice initially stemmed from the idea that everyone is driven by a section of our mind that is unconscious, some might even say instinctive. The constant challenges of our everyday lives cause us to react in ways that seem completely nonsensical until we open up this unconscious section of our minds.

Psychotherapists work on the belief that all of these thought processes step from childhood and other past experiences. Everything that makes us us comes from a selection of processes and beliefs that lie hidden until a psychotherapist manages to uncover them.

Life coaching

Although life coaching is a fairly new approach to talking therapy, it has grown in popularity over recent years because of the way it appears to change people's lives forever.

Life coaching lies somewhere between cognitive behavioural therapy and counselling, with a goal of uncovering the causes behind the ways in which you conduct your life. Once these causes have been discovered, the life coach begins to help you alter your thought processes and personal outlook.

Individuals are given a series of practical solutions which should help them develop a more positive outlook and improve their lives generally. Your coach will help you set yourself achievable goals by creating an optimistic atmosphere in which you can safely lay out your plans for the future.

Neuro-linguistic programming

Neuro-linguistic programming sounds incredibly complicated and futuristic, but its theory is surprisingly simple. This is a new science which starts with the belief that we need an understanding of how the brain works if we want a more positive experience of life. It's a system which works out why we act the way we do, and which thought process make us respond to different situations.

Therapists practicing neuro-linguistic programming will help you explore the sequences and maps that make up your thought processes, and identify which ones are stopping you from achieving your life goals. With these sequences as their guide, they can then identify sets of actions and exercises which will alter all of your unproductive brain programmes.

Group therapy

Talking about your personal feelings and experiences to a whole group rather than one trusted person can feel massively daunting. However, this is often an extremely effective type of talking therapy, so it's definitely worth considering. Be careful to pick the right group for you if you want to get all of the support you need. For guidance, you could talk to your GP or check the Internet, your local library or suggestions from friends.

Group therapy isn't simply a large group of people talking freely about their experiences – it'll be guided by a professional therapist who can instruct and guide the group in a calm, gentle way. But you will also benefit from hearing what other members of the group have to say, gaining new knowledge from their experiences and new support and friends from what was once a group of strangers.

Why should you consider group therapy?

When dealing with postnatal depression, it's absolutely vital that you know you are not alone. Finding an opportunity which allows you to share support and information in a group setting is often found to be a great way of improving self esteem. When you become part of a group, you get to feel as though you're part of something bigger than yourself, even when postnatal depression has caused you to feel alone, isolated or unusual.

It's important to be able to fully express your emotions and share what you're feeling. It can be a massive relief and reassurance to learn that the things you're feeling are completely normal, and that others in your group have felt or are feeling the same way. This can be especially helpful if anger becomes an issue as a result of your condition – it can be helpful to talk your frustrations through with an understanding group first, so that you don't end up just shouting at your partner out of the blue the next time you see them.

Done properly, a support group can be therapy at its very best, offering postnatal depression sufferers some of the vital medical and social support they need. They can be places to learn vital skills and build lasting friendships. There's no point in considering your condition to be a shameful secret that you need to deal with alone. There's strength in numbers, and the setting will give you unrivalled opportunities to share your thoughts, options and views.

Postnatal depression is an issue best worked through with family and friends, and in the best cases can lead to closer bonds between sufferers and those who have helped them. In some cases, members of groups will even learn not to resent or regret their postnatal depression, as it has offered such a great learning opportunity. Some therapists even encourage a feeling of shared learning through the use of group relaxation techniques.

They may even take on more of a coaching role, spurring on their group's progress by nurturing their goals and natural skills, and teaching new life skills. Attendees can learn to cope with things they never would have believed possible, and perfect skills they didn't know they already had. The trick is to acknowledge your condition before trying to change anything, as you can't make any progress without first doing this.

There's no use in taking on the role of 'victim' or living in denial. It's important to accept that the way you are feeling is a result of postnatal depression, and isn't simply the fault of someone close to you.

What have we learned?

The strongest way to work through mental health conditions such as postnatal depression is to talk things through. This will allow you to find your way to the other end by building all of the necessary bridges. The most basic form of talking therapy you can receive is a simple discussion with your family and friends. This can be incredibly helpful if you feel comfortable doing so, but some find it easier and more effective to talk openly to strangers, avoiding any feeling of judgement or emotional attachment.

Other forms of talking therapies include neuro-linguistic programming, psychotherapy and cognitive behavioural therapy. These all work in different ways, but the end goal is the same: To improve your mental health through talking. One option for talking therapy is basic counselling, which moves away from talking to your family and friends but will include similar conversations.

Some find it more helpful to join a support group, which can be a great way to help you feel understood and normal. Talking therapies can be used alongside any other treatments you receive, whether it's prescribed healthcare or an alternative therapy. In some cases, though, new mothers have found talking therapies so helpful that they haven't needed any other form of treatment.

Glossary

Aerobic exercise
Also known as 'cardio.' This is exercise which causes your heart to pump lots of oxygenated blood to your muscles by increasing your heart and breathing rates.

Antidepressant
A type of medication which is prescribed to alleviate the symptoms of depression.

Antipsychotic
A drug prescribed to relieve symptoms of mania, hypomania and psychosis.

Anxiety disorders
A group of psychological disorders characterized by unreasonable or excessive anxiety about certain aspects of life, with symptoms including palpitations, shortness of breath, or dizziness.

BAAM
British Association of Anger Management. Association specialising in providing support for stress, anger and conflict management. This support can take the form of individual support, workshops, seminars, bespoke packages and more.

Baby blues
This condition will make you feel unhappy, unable to cope and a little tearful for a few days, usually within 3-4 days of giving birth.

Bipolar disorder
A mental illness which is characterised by shifts between two extreme moods ('manic' and 'depressive' episodes).

Carer
The word used to describe anyone who cares for an elderly or ill person.

CBT
Cognitive Behavioural Therapy. This is a type of talking treatment whose aim is to alter unhelpful beliefs and thoughts which can lead to destructive behaviours and emotions.

Counselling
Another common talking treatment. Counselling involves providing a private, safe in which clients can talk about emotions they are experiencing and problems they are dealing with.

Depression
A long-lasting low mood, often with an absence of energy and enjoyment in previously favoured activities. Those experiencing persistent low moods may be diagnosed with clinical depression or major depressive disorder.

Diagnosis
Identification of a condition or illness through the examination of symptoms.

Endorphins
Neurotransmitters which are produced in response to stimuli such as fear, pain or stress. Endorphins mostly interact with receptors in parts of the brain responsible for controlling emotion and blocking pain.

GP
General Practitioner. This is a doctor who treats people in the wider community, also known as a family doctor.

Hallucination
An experience involving smelling, hearing or seeing something that isn't really there.

Health visitor
(SCPHN-HV) Registered and qualified midwives and nurses who have received extra qualifications and training to become specialist community public health nurses.

HRT
Hormone Replacement Therapy. A treatment where the patient received hormones to replace naturally occurring hormones with other hormones or supplement a lack of naturally occurring hormones.

Hypothyroidism
The condition which occurs when a person's thyroid gland fails to produce the required amount of the hormone thyroxine.

Insomnia
A condition characterised by persistent difficulty sleeping.

Interpersonal communication
Also known as face-to-face communication. This is how we exchange emotions, meanings and information through messages both verbal and non-verbal.

Labour
Word used to describe the process of childbirth, beginning with initial uterine contractions and ending with delivery.

Libido
Your sexual drive.

Mania
An abnormally positive, high mood.

Manic Depression
An older name for bipolar disorder. Though this term is still often used by the general public, it is seen as having negative connotations, and is no longer used in professional settings.

MAOI
Monoamine oxidase inhibitors. Rarely-prescribed antidepressants which work by acting on enzymes, rather than neurotransmitters.

Mental Health Foundation
A British charitable organisation which promotes research, information and improved services for those with mental health problems. The Foundation also incorporates the Foundation for People with Learning Disabilities.

Mental health support team

Also referred to as Community Mental Health Teams (CMHTs), this group supports people living in their community with serious or complex mental health problems.

Midwife

A professional who has been trained to assist women through childbirth.

Moclobemide

A newer type of MAOI which appears to cause fewer adverse effects than other similar medications. It's still advised that those taking this medication exercise great caution around certain medicines and foods.

Mood diary

This often comes in the form of a simple list of the ideas, behaviours and moods you experience each day that you may find worrying.

Mood disorder

Mental illnesses in which issues with an individual's mood are the main underlying feature. Bipolar disorder is an example.

Neurons

The basic working units of the brain. These are specially designed to communicate information between muscle, gland and nerve cells.

Neurotransmitters

Chemicals which transmit messages through the nerves between the body and the brain.

NICE

National Institute for Clinical Excellence. This is an independent organisation which is responsible for providing guidance nationwide on the treatment and prevention of illnesses and the promotion of good health in the United Kingdom.

Noradrenaline

Also known as norepinephrine. A neurotransmitter involved in alertness, formation and retrieval of memory, attention, vigilance and arousal.

OCD

Obsessive Compulsive Disorder. This is an anxiety disorder in which a person feels compelled to perform certain actions repeatedly to relieve intrusive thoughts or persistent fears.

Oestrogen

A group of hormones which promote the development and maintenance of female body characteristics.

OTC

Over the Counter. Any medicine which can be bought from a pharmacy without a prescription.

Paranoia

A feeling of persecution caused by delusional thinking.

Panic attack

A sudden, overwhelming experience of debilitating and acute anxiety.
Perfectionism
Inability to accept any standard short of perfection.

Postnatal Depression

A form of depression sometimes experienced by a mother after giving birth. This is usually as a result of a number of factors including psychological adjustments, fatigue and changes in hormone balance.

Pregnancy counselling

Talking treatments and other forms of psychological support received during pregnancy. These may include discussing any concerns you have about giving birth, CBT or straightforward counselling.

Preventative antidepressants

Antidepressants prescribed to a new mother in anticipation of postnatal depression, with an aim of preventing or reducing negative symptoms.

Progesterone

A hormone released by the Corpus Luteum to stimulate the uterus in preparation for pregnancy.

Psychiatrist

A doctor who specialises in mental illness.

Psycho-education

Teaching a patient and their family about the nature of their illness.

Psychological

Anything relating to the emotional or mental state of someone; of, arising from or affecting the mind.

Psychologist

Someone who is qualified to treat mental illness and study the human mind.

Psychosis

A condition in which the individual loses contact with reality.

PTSD

Post-Traumatic Stress Disorder. A condition characterised by persistent emotional and mental stress occurring as a result of injury or severe psychological shock.

Puerperal psychosis

A sudden loss of contact with external reality with hallucinations and confusion, often following childbirth.

SAD

Seasonal Affective Disorder. A mental illness which is believed to occur as a result of reduced sunlight in the winter months. SAD is a form of seasonal depression.

Self-care

A term used to describe any actions you may carry out in order to achieve improved mental and physical health.

Serotonin

A neurotransmitter which allows us to feel happiness.

Sleep hygiene

A selection of good patterns and practices which are vital in order to have a good quality of sleep at night and alertness during the day.

SNRIs

Serotonin-Norepinephrine Reuptake Inhibitors. One type of antidepressant, whose examples include Cymbalta and Effexor.

SSRIs

Selective Serotonin Reuptake Inhibitors. Another type of antidepressant, whose examples include Seroxat and Prozac.

Support group

A formal meeting with a group of other people in a similar situation to you. This is sometimes called 'peer support'.

Talking therapy

Treatment for mental health issues which involves therapy and discussion, either along with or instead of medication. Examples include CBT and counselling.

Thyroid disease

A condition often occurring as a result of pregnancy, with symptoms including changes in weight, low mood and extreme fatigue.

Traumatic birth

A traumatic or distressing birth experience. This can include things like very long or very quick, painful labours, excessive levels of intervention or the birth of an injured baby.
Find more information on the Birth Trauma Association's website (www.birthtraumaassociation.org.uk/help-support/what-is-birth-trauma)

Tricyclic

An older type of antidepressant, which has now been replaced by SSRIs and SNRIs in most cases.

Unipolar

Another name for major depressive disorder.

Warning signs

Early indicators that someone may be at risk of developing the condition. For postnatal depression, these may include depression, isolation or obsessive behaviours.

Withdrawal symptoms

The horrible emotional and physical reaction which is experienced when someone stops taking an addictive substance.

Help List

Association for Postnatal Illness (APNI)
145 Dawes Road, Fulham, London, SW6 7EB
Tel: 020 7386 0868
www.apni.org
A well-established charitable organisation, they aim to support sufferers, increase knowledge about the condition and promote ongoing research into the causes of postnatal depression. APNI have a very helpful website with a variety of information leaflets.

Birth Trauma Association (BTA)
PO Box 671, Ipswich, Suffolk, IP1 9AT
www.birthtraumaassociation.org.uk
BTA supports all women who have had a traumatic birth experience.

Depression Alliance
20 Great Dover Street, London, SE1 4LX
Tel: 0845 123 23 20
information@depressionalliance.org
www.depressionalliance.org
A leading UK charity which aims to raise awareness of depression and improve public services and support for sufferers.

Homestart
Tel: 0800 068 63 68
www.home-start.org.uk
Homestart is a national treasure! They provide trained volunteers who will visit homes on a regular basis to relieve and support the mothers of babies and young children.

Meet a Mum Association (MAMA)
54 Lillington Road, Radstock, BA3 3NR
Tel: 0845 120 3746 (helpline, Monday to Friday, 7-10pm)
MAMA provides friendship and support networks for mothers with postnatal depression. Their website is very informative.

MIND

PO Box 277, Manchester, M60 3XN

Tel: 0845 766 0163 (helpline)

info@mind.org.uk

www.mind.org.uk

MIND addresses all forms of mental illness and offers some invaluable helpline services.

NaPro Technology

www.naprotechnology.com

Features a good page dedicated to postnatal depression and Dr Katharina Dalton.

National Childbirth Trust (NCT)

Tel: 0300 330 0772 (pregnancy and birth line)

Tel: 0300 330 0771 (breastfeeding line)

Tel: 0300 330 0773 (postnatal line)

Tel: 0300 330 0770 (enquiries line)

Tel: 0300 330 0774 (shared experiences line)

www.nctpregnancyandbabycare.com

NCT help over a million mums and dads each year through pregnancy, birth and early days of parenthood. They offer antenatal and postnatal courses, local support and reliable information to help all parents.

Natural Progesterone Advisory Network

www.natural-progesterone-advisory-network.com

A comprehensive insight into the issue of hormone replacement as a treatment for postnatal depression.

Netmums

www.netmums.co.uk

A great parenting resource with forums. They directly address and support members suffering with postnatal depression.

Parentline Plus

Tel: 0808 800 222 (helpline)

www.parentlineplus.org.uk

Parenting guidance and advice tailor-made for mothers and fathers.

Perinatal Illness – UK

PO Box 49769, London, WC1H 9WH

deb@pni-uk.com

www.pni-uk.com

A charity which addresses antenatal and postnatal illnesses, puerperal psychosis and birth trauma.

PND Support

Tel: 800 043 2031 (helpline, Monday to Friday, 9am-7pm)

help@pndsupport.co.uk

www.pndsupport.co.uk

A warm and personal resource run by two former sufferers of postnatal depression.

Progesterone Link

www.progesteronelink.com

You can find some information about progesterone therapy on this website.

Relate

Tel: 0300 100 1234

www.relate.org.uk

Relate are the country's largest provider of relationship support – find more about the services they offer and where they're located via the website.

Samaritans

Chris, PO Box 9090, Stirling, FK8 2SA

Tel: 08457 90 90 90

jo@samaritans.org

www.samaritans.org

This charity is a confidential source of emotional support.

SANEline

1st Floor Cityside House, 40 Adler Street London E1 1EE

Tel: 0845 767 8000 (helpline)

www.sane.org.uk

A far-reaching organisation which raises awareness, assists research and provides help and information for people with mental health issues.